Mental Health: Intervention Skills for the Emergency Services

Tricia Scott

Editor

Mental Health: Intervention Skills for the Emergency Services

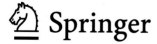 Springer

Editor
Tricia Scott 🆔
Middlesbrough, UK

ISBN 978-3-031-20346-6   ISBN 978-3-031-20347-3   (eBook)
https://doi.org/10.1007/978-3-031-20347-3

This Springer imprint is published by the registered company Springer Nature Switzerland AG
The registered company address is: Gewerbestrasse 11, 6330 Cham, Switzerland

Foreword

This teaching text has brought together a range of expertise to address issues central to the mental health and welfare of patients and emergency care fields. The work is thoughtful, and every attempt is made to centre the patient in each chapter to provide the golden thread which galvanises the book. People who experience the emergency pathway during mental health crisis may experience heightened emotion, feel out of control, become isolated, sometimes fearing judgemental opinion due to negative attitudes from others. This means that emergency care practitioners and allied emergency services personnel who support them need to understand their own attitudes toward mental ill-health and to develop skills which enable them to recognise deep pain and vulnerability in another person and to willingly provide supportive measures.

Dr Scott rightly begins the book by honouring those people who truly bear the risk of poor services, the patients, people and their families with lived experience of a mental health condition, many of whom bear the real and metaphorical scars of distress and lack of support. There is no doubt, people with lived experience of mental illness have not always received the most appropriate help to meet their needs, especially at the time they needed it the most, i.e. when they were in crisis. There are a number of factors that contribute to this, as is very well mapped in this book, and ultimately, patients and staff often come away from urgent and emergency response scenarios feeling like it has been a challenge which has not necessarily produced the most beneficial of outcomes for the patient or their family.

The book then takes us through a range of scenarios and considerations using an all-age approach and so you will learn about the children and young people's experiences alongside adults and older adults. These pages discuss the incidence and nature of mental health presentations, legislation, policy and contemporary research; it also incorporates case studies and provides bullet points for reflection and inspires the reader with a real sense of what could be possible if best practice could be applied across the urgent and emergency care system. Chapter authors provide both an understanding of the difficulties and complexities involved in caring for people in crisis within the emergency pathway whilst also offering hope and ideas for what could be handled better. This book will challenge emergency care practitioners and allied emergency services to do better by developing contemporary and well-researched evidence-based interventions.

Centre for Mental Health   Sarah Hughes
London, UK

Acknowledgement

This book is dedicated to the many people who have lived through painful mental health crisis and who have taught us as emergency services and allied health personnel. People who were living with some extremely distressing symptoms of mental ill-health, distorted cognitions, anxiety, depression and suicidal ideation. To support people in mental health crisis is a privilege, and it takes a long time to understand the complexities involved as we try to interpret their behaviour and respond effectively to each situation. One particular aspect I remember being taught during my initial mental health nurse training is that there is a person inside who is desperately trying to get back to a state of calm.

As a Mental Health Nurse and Registered Adult Nurse working in the Emergency Department, I recall a man in his late thirties who arrived by ambulance with 'epileptic fits'. I sensed some kind of incongruity, and something didn't sit well with me. This was because the 'fits' didn't seem to follow the usual tonic-clonic presentation and further, with none of the usual urinary incontinence. That's OK, we know that there are many types of fits. As the team were about to administer medicines to suppress these 'fits', I took the bold but risky step of asking everyone to leave the room so I could talk with him. They left then I gently asked the man if they were real fits and if there was anything else going on that could be contributing to his situation. After a momentary pause, he became immensely tearful and fretful, he seemed to need space and time to articulate what was distressing him: responsibility for his demanding work, his unhappiness with his home life, the kids, money worries, this…that…everything! After the doctor was updated, stress and anxiety became the actual diagnosis and the man left the department with a new sense of hope after having his feelings validated through a focused conversation.

I learned two things that day first, to read the situation because things are not always what they seem so emergency practitioners should caution against hasty decisions and diagnoses when there may be more going on. Second, the power of authentic conversation between emergency services practitioners and patients can lead to new hope that life may become a little easier for them after working through a cathartic experience. Supporting someone during overwhelming crisis can be tough, but by untangling emotions and recognising that choices are available may be the first step in returning to our 'centre' and what anchors us. Emergency practitioner intuition offers a major influence on our actions and all the policies and procedures in the world cannot replace the gut feeling that something simply doesn't add up. This feature of mental health encounters should not be ignored. Intuition tends to lead to risk taking, as we read between the lines to access the metanarrative and to question whether their words convey true meaning and intent. In essence, is the person safe or at risk of deepening crisis, self-harm, suicide?

I dedicate this book to all those people who have shaped our thinking about mental health in emergency care.

Contents

Mental Health as a Societal Concept Impacting on Emergency Care

Tricia Scott

1   Introduction

Mental health as a societal concept which needs to be addressed has been gathering momentum in the past decade. This is due to a number of policy drivers. The World Health Organisation (WHO) included mental health as one of the Sustainable Development Goals stating how "…depression is one of the leading causes of disability. Suicide is the second leading cause of death among 15-29-year-olds. People with severe mental health conditions die prematurely—as much as two decades early—due to preventable physical conditions" [1]. In 2019 the WHO launched the WHO Special Initiative for Mental Health (2019–2023): Universal Health Coverage for Mental Health to ensure access to appropriate mental health care in 12 priority countries. This was because, despite progress, mental health conditions are associated with severe human rights violations, discrimination and stigma.

Recently, COVID-19 further impacted on population health as the "…COVID-19 pandemic triggers 25% increase in prevalence of anxiety and depression worldwide" [2] and, as Dr. Tedros Adhanom Ghebreyesus, WHO Director General stated, such an increase suggests, "The information we have now about the impact of COVID-19 on the world's mental health is just the tip of the iceberg". Such an increase means, "This is a wake-up call to all countries to pay more attention to mental health and do a better job of supporting their populations' mental health". COVID-19 response plans need to accommodate the should provide support measures; however, major gaps remain in many countries. In all, the most recent Health Atlas declared on average only just over 2% of their health budget was devoted to mental health in 2020, which contributed to the global shortage in mental health services. Such historical underinvestment has largely contributed to the current state

T. Scott (✉)
Independent Education and Research Consultant, North Yorkshire, UK

T. Scott (ed.), *Mental Health: Intervention Skills for the Emergency Services*,
https://doi.org/10.1007/978-3-031-20347-3_1

of affairs, and countries must act urgently to prioritise mental health services and access to the same.

In the European context, Stewart [3] reported that the most commonly diagnosed mental health diseases include depression, generalised anxiety and eating disorders, whereby the affected person feels sad and/or down, withdraws from social life and experiences anger, substance abuse and suicidal thoughts. Adding to the complexity of the experience, about 25% of the population in many European countries reported that they suffered from at least one mental health condition, anxiety disorders being slightly higher than depression. Compounding factors such as substance use may add to the complexity of treatment and support with the need for additional structures to be arranged to help that person manage their situation.

In the UK context the Office for National Statistics [4] January figures report that "1.49 million people were in contact with mental health services, at the end of December. The majority of these (1,007,387) were in contact with adult services" and "355,807 people were in contact with children and young people's mental health services, at the end of December". Further, "175,083 people were in contact with learning disabilities and autism services, at the end of December" and "20,894 people were subject to the Mental Health Act, including 15,647 people detained in hospital, at the end of December" [5]. These seem disturbing statistics; however, statistics alone, whilst important indicators of the scale of the problem and patterns of access do not reflect or explain the complexity and nuances of the mental health, mental ill-health and mental health crisis experience. That is very much brought to life through the reflections and narratives of the people affected so it is important that we hear their stories and listen to their plight, help people to manage their condition and work responsively with them and their families towards a solution to calm their situation. Locally, mental health is gaining increasing public attention through the work of mental health charities which capitalise on social media to get their message across, e.g. the HRH Heads Together Campaign. Such efforts encourage people from all walks of life to become more receptive to the notion that every family is affected by mental health issues, so there may indeed be a greater awareness of the effects on family members who support someone who is experiencing, e.g. depression, anxiety or a psychotic episode.

Causative factors vary such as relationship breakdown, work pressures, geographical detachment from families as well as chemical and hormonal imbalance and various theories exist to explain the aetiology of mental ill-health. Theoretical concepts and explanations of the potential aetiology of mental illness derive from psychodynamic, behavioural, cognitive, social, humanistic and biological theories [6]. Whilst theoretical understanding provides an important framework, any attempt to address the societal problem means that action is needed, so it is interesting to note how UK local authority election candidates are currently focusing their manifesto on the following key strategies: reducing poverty, improving the environment, supporting the best start in life and ensuring access to quality services. Whilst the UK government White Paper aims to level up specific sectors such as economic disparities, devolution, digital connectivity and housing, there is little reference to what impact these will have on the mental health of the population [7]. The final report of the Commission for Equality in Mental Health [8] finds that mental health inequalities mirror wider economic and social inequalities and creates sharp social divisions so that many people experience three times the risk of mental ill-health. The emergency services support many of these people through crisis, and action is needed to address the recurrent problem of stigmatised attitudes, fragmented services and a lack of support. There is a clear need to drive change by improving policy and practice, to work at building communities and, most importantly, to do so through the voices of those who live with mental health issues.

The International Classification of Diseases DSM 5 was updated in 2022 to the DSM 5-TR edition. Recent editions of the DSM have received praise for trying to standardise psychiatric diagnosis based on empirical evidence yet concurrently generated controversy and criticism and a crisis in confidence in the reliability and validity of many diagnoses. Common assumptions and dated interpretations of autism provide a good example of societal misinterpretation particularly when considering the difference between dated assumptions about a linear "autism spectrum" which comprises two polarities and which can result in damaging misattribution, invalidation, exclusion and othering. Instead, autism may comprise multiple elements which may or may not be experienced by different individuals, e.g. sensory sensitivities or repetitive behaviours. Most important then is to consider the person as a human being by acknowledging their difficulties when trying to get by in a society which can at best be judgemental and reactionary and to help them return to a state of calm, recover and regain balance so they may make important decisions for themselves about their own care especially when experiencing the fast-paced emergency milieu.

2   The Emergency Care Field

Specific to this book is the urgent and emergency care field which is known to be a highly emotionally charged environment characterised by time-sensitive algorithms and immediate decision-making to direct people to the most appropriate pathway to prevent deterioration. However, whilst a number of major improvements have been made, e.g. mental health liaison or paramedic/mental health nurse teams and policing reform, there is indeed scope for further investment and enhancement in the area of mental health. The doctrine of emergency medicine has traditionally prioritised the physical aspects of patient assessment and treatment, so it is unsurprising that nursing staff sense a lack of relevant training on mental health care which leaves them feeling unprepared to care for their patients effectively including how to support young people, patients who self-harm, autism and/or learning disability. It may therefore be helpful to practitioners to refer to the various guidelines published by the Royal College of Emergency Medicine and to incorporate the recommendations into practice, e.g., the Mental Health Toolkit [9] the Mental Capacity Act Guideline [10] and position statements such as *ED doctors performing MHA assessments in England and Wales* [11].

Emergency practitioners have necessarily been self-critical of previous intolerance of patients presenting with mental health needs and embrace the notion that (a) we should be much more tolerant of people who display signs and symptoms of mental ill-health and (b) mental ill-health is increasingly recognised among the emergency practitioner community itself, as a high-stress occupational group. To do so we must look inward at our own shortcomings and consider more effective ways to respond to someone experiencing mental crisis and to authentically support both patients and colleagues. Whatever the aetiology, mental ill-health is very much a personal experience as the person affected juggles the anguish of their condition and their fear of, e.g. depression, paranoia, hallucinations, delusions, hypomania or suicidal ideation. It is also a family experience as they try to understand what their loved one is going through and, beyond first presentations, often feel they may be unable to cope with a further episode of instability. Staff tend to rely heavily on the information and support of families and Chap. 2 "Learning Disability and Sensory Processing Conditions" suggests some helpful indicators in this regard. Of course, not all people experiencing mental health instability have a devoted and caring family to cushion them in crisis. Many live in isolation, fear, despair and hopelessness compounded by quite difficult personal circumstances such as being homeless, sofa surfing, being out of work or, indeed, following bereavement. It is known that the critical combination of severe depression and hopelessness creates the ingredients for a suicide attempt, yet the emergency system continues to use simplistic and inadequate measures to assess suicidal ideation and risk. Shortfalls within the Manchester Triage System need urgent attention to save lives.

It is vital that we treat people within the emergency pathway with dignity and respect, so it is interesting to consider the words we select when describing people who attend with mental health conditions. A negative narrative seems to have emerged through the use of words such as "challenging", "disruptive", "unpredictable" "aggressive" or "demanding" and such words appear in nursing reports contributing to a negative discourse, perpetuating fears associated with mental health presentations and stigmatising and marginalising this patient cohort [12]. So, in light of the above lack of awareness which can result in misinterpretation and misattribution, how equipped do emergency practitioners feel about approaching and assessing people who display symptoms of mental ill-health? Whilst some people present with fairly innocuous symptoms, others may seem reasonably alert and lucid on first contact then during conversation may reveal some quite distorted thought processes, e.g. paranoia, hallucinations (visual, auditory, tactile) and/or delusions. The ability of a practitioner to recognise these symptoms and respond effectively with authenticity and in compliance with mental health and human rights legislation begs questions about the quality of their training and preparation for role. Indeed, physical health outcomes are poorer, and suicidal risk is increased, where depression, anxiety and other mental health conditions are unmanaged. Additionally, trauma-informed services acknowledge the strong link between trauma and subsequent mental illness. So, what does that mean to the emergency practitioner and allied emergency services? It means that public services need to be trauma-informed and to tread carefully and sensitively when supporting someone who has suffered violating experiences, e.g. domestic and sexual exploitation or assault, and to remember that it is essential that they feel welcomed within the emergency pathway as a genuine "place of safety".

The Care Quality Commission Report [13] highlighted how ED staff feel unsupported and unprepared to care for their patients' mental health needs, so, for staff to provide high-quality care for their patients, appropriate training is necessary to enhance competence and confidence. Indeed, some staff viewed their mental health support role as outside of their remit relying heavily on psychiatry teams to handle this aspect. The CQC found that mental health training for staff varied, which was often limited to mandatory e-learning that focused on legislation including the Mental Capacity Act 2005 and Deprivation of Liberty Safeguards, but not the Mental Health Act 1983. Discharge summaries routinely requested depression screening to be carried out by general practitioners, yet medical teams should be able to have a holistic conversation with patients who are worried or showing signs of depression (p. 21).

How attentive and empathic a practitioner remains is of huge benefit to the person who is living through crisis because this helps to build trust. As an emergency practitioner, being aware of one's own posturing, spatiality, pitch and tone of voice, monitoring expressions of bias and judgemental projections are so important in the formation of a therapeutic interaction with someone who is feeling at their lowest or is experiencing thought disturbance. Indeed, the need to remain mute and unresponsive should also be respected as this may be symptomatic of a deep and painful depression. In social interaction terms, the patient's reaction may provide the "mirror within", the reflection of the emergency practitioner's own projections. So, it is helpful for the emergency practitioner to remain calm, non-judgemental, compassionate and sincere about the situation that person is living through and the anguish they may be expressing. These responses provide lasting impressions. De-escalation involves using calming measures to avoid overstimulation so reducing noise, lights, and presence of too many people, talking the person down to a manageably calm state and empowering the person to exercise agency through choice are essential steps in creating a therapeutic milieu. The core values of a person-centred health service which treats its emergency patients with dignity and compassion should be upheld.

3   New Approaches

The legislative framework for mental health support undergoes regular refinement to ensure that people experiencing mental instability are fully supported and their liberty protected. Throughout the book reference will be made to various pieces of legislation in particular the Mental Health Act and the Mental Capacity Act, and attention is drawn to proposals for legislative change. Chapter 4 "Police Custody Officer" summarises some key legislative changes to support people in custody who may be experiencing mental disturbance and to direct them to the most appropriate location for their needs. It is encouraging then to note that nowadays people in mental health crisis are less likely to be taken to a police cell as a place of safety and more likely be directed to a health facility. One recent major development consists of the Mental Health Liaison Team which facilitates assessment and support by the most appropriate specialists early in the emergency pathway (Chap. 6 "Mental Health Liaison Team").

The Crisis Care Concordat (CCC, 2014) was launched which involves multi-agency collaboration to action the best solution for the patient, and this approach moves away from the traditional boundaries of practice to embrace a multi-agency, multi-professional collaborative approach. This is a particularly helpful transition considering mind/body relevance central to mental health: mind having causal relevance on behaviour through highly interconnected systems. Parity of esteem between physical and psychological health is highlighted later in the book. Chapter 2 "Learning Disability and Sensory Processing Conditions" draws on the experiences of people who live with a learning disability some of whom may also have an autistic condition. The fact that people who have a learning disability are likely to die 20 years earlier than the rest of the population and due to avoidable causes brings sharp focus to the need to closely examine our systems and processes to ensure that people with a LD/autism are comprehensively assessed within the emergency pathway. It is therefore critical that every patient contact matters so that a person who experiences mental health crisis is treated with the same urgency as those with physical health needs.

4   Where to Find Help

An argument exists that lengthy waiting times for psychological services and an underdeveloped range of alternative care pathways mean patients default to an emergency pathway due to a build up to crisis point. Social value of mental health patients in the emergency pathway is apparent, e.g. paramedics are frequently the first point of contact for people experiencing mental health crisis in the community (Chap. 3 "Paramedic"). In the past, the social value of the patient may have impacted negatively on patient care and treatment due to them being considered a distraction from "real" emergency care problems, usually life- or limb-threatening physical presentations. For people who live with autism, differences in sensory processing can be quite painful for the autistic person and in some situations may induce autistic meltdown as a reaction to extremely stressful situations such as emergency department attendance (Chap. 2 "Learning Disability and Sensory Processing Conditions"). Challenging behaviours add to the complexity of care and can also risk the personal safety of the emergency professionals involved which is of particular concern for practitioners who must establish a differential diagnosis, for example, in the case of a person sustaining a head injury influenced by alcohol consumption.

Mental health crisis may affect anyone regardless of social demographic, so it is helpful to consider the impact on different patient groups, e.g. children and young people (Chap. 8 "Children and Young Peoples' Services") as well as older adults (Chap. 9 "Older People Mental Health") and, indeed, older old. Of relevance is the need to retain person-centredness, dignity and choice whilst the person is living through a difficult situation such as the older adult who has dementia and who has sustained an injury after a fall which brings them in contact with emergency services. Indeed, poly-morbidity and polypharmacy associated with older people provide additional complexity when assessing and planning care for someone in contact with the emergency services who may be older and mentally ill. The physical aspects of their care need to be thoroughly assessed as they may live with additional physical health problems, e.g. poor diet and nutrition, altered bowel habits, poor dental hygiene, limited health screening and the effects of longer-term medication, particularly psychotropic medication.

One particularly important aspect of emergency care for people experiencing mental ill-health concerns the attempt to take one's own life through an overdose. The public generally do not understand that the narrow therapeutic range of some drugs means that in overdose they may be sufficient to unintentionally kill you whilst other drugs may have a much lower toxicity threshold which may render them safer in overdose. Chapter 10 "Toxicology in Parasuicide" acknowledges that the interval between ingestion/exposure and treatment is critical to establish because accurate timelines determine treatment regimes. Further, there is limited awareness of the fact that few antidotes exist for specific substances, and, therefore, symptomatic treatment may be necessary. Intentionality is key to an accurate mental health assessment and diagnosis which paves the way for accurate treatment and support. However, continued risk assessment and safety of the patient are imperative whilst the patient remains in hospital. Knowledge of various clusters of symptoms associated with a specific toxicity state, otherwise known as toxidrome, is helpful to the practitioner especially when the patient is unable or unwilling to state what they have deliberately ingested. However, this knowledge is recorded as an adjunct to TOXBASE® confirmation and advice. Practitioners should become aware of the role and contact details for the National Poisons Information Service.

This chapter concludes by encouraging emergency services practitioners to become more familiar with the nuances of the vast array of mental health presentations that they could encounter on a daily basis and to adapt one's approach to facilitate a therapeutic and meaningful communication which is calming and helpful. Each chapter takes on a specific emergency discipline and discusses situations of relevance, and occasional scenarios highlight some quite tricky dilemmas and suggest strategies for how staff might respond offering concluding learning points to enable understanding and reflection on personal practice.

References

1. World Health Organization. Mental Health. 2022. https://www.who.int/health-topics/mental-health#tab=tab_1
2. Brunier A. COVID-19 pandemic triggers 25% increase in prevalence of anxiety and depression worldwide. News release. 2nd March 2022. 2022. https://www.who.int/news/item/02-03-2022-covid-19-pandemic-triggers-25-increase-in-prevalence-of-anxiety-and-depression-worldwide

3. Stewart C. Statista. Mental health in Europe - statistics & facts 31st May 2021. 2021. https://www.statista.com/topics/7916/mental-health-in-europe/#dossierKeyfigures

4. Office for National Statistics. Mental health services monthly statistics, performance December 2021, provisional January 2022. 2022. https://digital.nhs.uk/data-and-information/publications/statistical/mental-health-services-monthly-statistics/performance-december-2021-provisional-january-2022

5. NHS Digital. Mental health services monthly statistics, Performance December 2021, Provisional January 2022. 2022. https://digital.nhs.uk/data-and-information/publications/statistical/mental-health-services-monthly-statistics/performance-december-2021-provisional-january-2022

6. O'Regan PH. Theories of mental health and illness: psychodynamic, social, cognitive, behavioral, humanistic, and biological influences (chapter 10). In: Nurse Key. 2017. https://nursekey.com/theories-of-mental-health-and-illness-psychodynamic-social-cognitive-behavioral-humanistic-and-biological-influences/

7. Bell A. Levelling Up the UK: what does it mean for mental health? Centre for Mental Health. 2022. https://www.centreformentalhealth.org.uk/blogs/levelling-uk-what-does-it-mean-mental-health

8. Centre for Mental Health Commission for Equality in Mental Health. Mental health for all? The final report of the Commission for Equality in Mental Health. 2020. https://www.centreformentalhealth.org.uk/sites/default/files/publication/download/Commission_FinalReport_updated.pdf

9. Royal College of Emergency Medicine. Mental Health in Emergency Departments: a toolkit for improving care. 2022. https://rcem.ac.uk/wp-content/uploads/2022/02/Mental_Health_Toolkit_Feb_2022_Update.pdf

10. Royal College of Emergency Medicine. The Mental Capacity Act in Emergency Medicine Practice. 2017. https://rcem.ac.uk/wp-content/uploads/2021/10/RCEM_Mental_Capacity_Act_in_EM_Practice_Feb2017.pdf

11. Royal College of Emergency Medicine. Position Statement: ED Doctors performing Mental Health Act assessments in England and Wales. 2020. https://res.cloudinary.com/studio-republic/images/v1635416629/ED_Doctors_Performing_MHA_Assessments_in_England_and_Wales_Position_Statement/ED_Doctors_Performing_MHA_Assessments_in_England_and_Wales_Position_Statement.pdf?_i=AA

12. Scott T. It's vital we treat people presenting at ED with mental health issues with care. Emerg Nurse. 2020;28(2):5. https://doi.org/10.7748/en.28.2.5.s1.

13. Care Quality Commission. Assessment of mental health services in acute trusts programme Report: How are people's mental health needs met in acute hospitals, and how can this be improved? 2020. https://www.cqc.org.uk/sites/default/files/20201016b_AMSAT_report.pdf

Learning Disability and Autistic Spectrum Conditions

Liz Herrieven

1 Background and Introduction

1.1 Learning Disability

What exactly is a learning disability (LD)? According to Mencap [1], it is "…a reduced intellectual ability and difficulty with everyday activities which affects someone for their whole life. People with LD tend to take longer to learn and may need support to develop new skills, understand complicated information and interact with other people". This is different to a learning *difficulty*, which does not affect intellect, but still makes learning more challenging, for example dyslexia or attention deficit hyperactivity disorder. The causes of LD are many and varied, ranging from genetic or chromosomal anomalies to birth injuries, neonatal sepsis or childhood trauma, for example but all affect the developing brain. Some people with a LD may have other associated physical conditions, such as those with Down syndrome, whilst others may not. A learning disability may affect one particular area of learning, such as auditory learning for example, with relative strengths in other areas such as visual learning, or it may be more general, affecting many different areas of learning. Learning disabilities are often categorised as mild, moderate or severe, the latter may sometimes also be called profound. They may coexist with autism (which will be discussed in the sensory processing section later in this chapter), which is not itself a learning disability but which can also affect the way a person is able to interpret and navigate the world around them [2].

There are about 1.5 million people living with LD in the UK comprising 2.16% adults and 2.5% children [3], so an emergency department (ED)

L. Herrieven (✉)
Emergency Department, Sheffield Children's Hospital, Sheffield, UK
e-mail: elizabeth.herrieven@nhs.net

© The Author(s), under exclusive license to Springer Nature
Switzerland AG 2023
T. Scott (ed.), *Mental Health: Intervention Skills for the Emergency Services*,
https://doi.org/10.1007/978-3-031-20347-3_2

9

receiving 200 patients a day could reasonably expect to see about 4 or 5 patients with LD each day. Some of these disabilities will be mild, and not obvious to ED staff, whilst others may provide significant challenges to both staff and the patient and family.

Of course, that four or five patients per day is purely an estimate. Many people with LD will have other conditions, often as a result of the cause of their LD for example people with Down syndrome, one of the most common causes of LD, may also have congenital cardiac disease, coeliac disease, or hypothyroidism, and people with LD secondary to a hypoxic brain injury may also have epilepsy. That four or five per day may actually be higher, so all ED staff need to know how best to care for patients with LD, whatever emergency they may present with.

People with a LD are likely to die on average 20 years earlier than people without a LD [4]. The Learning Disability Mortality Review (LeDeR) [5], found significant issues with the care of patients with LD prior to their deaths. People with LD are more likely to die due to an avoidable cause of death than those without LD, in particular a cause of death which ought to be treatable, such as pneumonia or sepsis. There are many factors behind this and, in order to best care for patients with LD in the ED, it is important to understand some of them. This chapter aims to explore these factors and to identify some of the ways ED practitioners can improve care for patients with LD.

Anne Hunt, who has worked as Lead Nurse for Sepsis at East and North Hertfordshire NHS Trust, is an excellent example of how healthcare professionals can do this. She understood that sepsis was not always recognised [6], especially in patients with LD, so set out to raise awareness of the condition amongst these patients and their families, distributing information in a format which was easy to read and understand. She worked alongside providers of LD services to explore ways of sharing information, including the utility of "soft signs," which we will talk more about shortly. She also worked with health professionals to identify reasons for late diagnosis, improve knowledge and education regarding LD and promote best practices.

2   Patient Factors

Some of the factors which contribute to the differences in morbidity and mortality are related to intrinsic differences in the patients themselves. Patients with LD, by definition, face challenges when it comes to everyday tasks. Those tasks will include things such as understanding how to stay healthy, being able to choose and prepare nutritious food and to take part in exercise, knowing what to do and who to contact when feeling unwell, being able to convey information about how they are feeling, remembering to take medication and so on, even before we consider elements such as an increased likelihood of comorbidities and polypharmacy. It may feel as though we, as ED professionals, cannot do much about these patient-related factors, but actually, we are in a good position to support our patients in many of these areas. Simple things such as providing health information in an easy read [7] format or a dossette box for medications can make a huge difference.

3   Communication

Communication is vitally important in all healthcare interactions, but it becomes even more so if your patient has a LD, and it can make the difference between getting the right outcome for your patient and completely missing the mark. First, we need to recognise that a person's ability to communicate does not always give an indication of their level of understanding. Someone might be able to speak very well, but be unable to understand the instructions or questions with which they are faced. Alternatively, someone may not be able to communicate verbally, but may be able to understand very clearly what is being said to them and, more importantly, about them within earshot by others. We also need to recognise that communication is a two-way process and that we, as healthcare professionals, can have a big impact on not only how we communicate and are understood, but also how we ourselves are able to understand others.

For some, good communication may be as simple as speaking slowly, clearly, avoiding medical jargon, and ensuring that our environment is quiet and without distraction. For others, we may need to find alternative ways to communicate. A large proportion of communication is non-verbal, so it is sometimes helpful if we, as emergency department practitioners, ask ourselves what our body language is conveying to our patients and how we might use that body language to help reassure and comfort. This may mean sitting down at the same level as the patient when talking with them which is less threatening. Similarly, it is important to interpret what the patient is trying to say through their body language, demeaner, posturing and eye contact. Consider those behaviours which create barriers (barrier signs, e.g. arms folded across chest) and those which may encourage a more comfortable dynamic (tie signs, e.g. turning towards the person to speak).

It is important to consider whether gesture, or even sign language, may help with our communication. Many people with LD use some form of sign-augmented communication, such as Makaton [8]. This visual representation of spoken words can help to support those who have difficulty with auditory memory, hearing or understanding. Even without a formal sign language, gestures can help to clarify things when used alongside verbal communication. Other ways to support the spoken word include the use of symbols or pictures, such as PECS [9]. These can be used in a variety of ways. An ED practitioner may, for example use a board of PECS symbols to point out interventions which may happen, or a patient may use the symbols to explain symptoms such as pain or vomiting. Photos or simple diagrams can be used in a similar way. Pre-prepared boards or cards can be invaluable, but if these are not available then pointing to body parts or equipment to provide a visual support to verbal information can also be useful.

Not only do we need to ensure the information we give is clear, but we also need to make every attempt to listen to and acknowledge what our patients are saying. Do we need help with understanding signs, or even words spoken with difficulty? Family and carers may be able to understand our patients more easily than we can. We need to remember to give our patients an opportunity to communicate with us and enough time to respond to us to enable thought processing during what may be an overwhelming experience. Some patients, for example those with Down syndrome, may have an auditory processing delay. It can take several seconds for the steps which others take for granted, to occur in that a sound has to travel to the inner ear, be converted to an electrical signal, make its way to the right area of the brain to be understood and a reply formulated; that reply then needs to travel, via nerve conduction, to the muscles responsible for facial movements and breathing and to the vocal cords, and then that reply has to be produced as a series of sounds. This all becomes more difficult and takes longer if you have glue ear, a sensorineural hearing problem, auditory memory issues, delayed understanding, a smaller vocabulary, and weaker muscles. Of significance, hearing loss has a tenfold higher incidence among children with LD and autism and glue ear is a particularly associated condition [10] so practitioners need to assess the most helpful form of communication.

4   Diagnostic Overshadowing

Diagnostic overshadowing is a huge problem for patients with complex conditions, LD or autism. This occurs when a person already has a pre-existing diagnosis, and any new symptoms or signs are put down to this same diagnosis without the healthcare professional considering other possible causes. For example, a child with Down syndrome might present as being quiet and floppy and the clinician may decide that this is due to the child having Down syndrome without looking for other causes, such as possible sepsis. Or an autistic person may present as being quite anxious and agitated, perhaps with repetitive hand movements, and the clinician may decide that this is just because he/she is autistic, without considering whether he/she may be in pain or feeling unwell.

Bias can be very difficult to avoid in healthcare and the only real way to avoid diagnostic overshadowing is to recognise your susceptibility to it, put your initial thoughts to one side and to actively consider other diagnoses. An accurate history is vital and you may need to gather a collateral history from family and carers also. They can offer helpful information to know more about what the patient is like when they are well and how they may appear when ill. Clinical examination should be thorough, as for any other patient, but the practitioner may need to take a little more time for the assessment to be carried out in a pragmatic and opportunistic way. Observational skills can be key, particularly when assessing patients who are unable to cooperate with the instructions associated with neurological or joint examinations, for example.

5   Sensory Processing Issues

Sensory processing issues are relatively common amongst people with LD, particularly those with Down syndrome or who also happens to be autistic. People who live with Autistic Spectrum Conditions (ASC) experience the world in a different way to neurotypical people and altered sensory processing is a key feature.

ASC is a lifelong developmental disability which affects how a person communicates and interacts with the world around them. Persistent difficulties concern social interaction, communication and stereotypic behaviours such as rigidity and repetition, resistance to change or restricted interests [11]. For some, anxiety is exacerbated by intolerance of uncertainty, for example in situations in which they do not know what is going to happen nor how long that uncertainty is likely to last. Emergency treatment in an unfamiliar clinical environment may add to their inability to cope and can, for some, lead to autistic meltdown (to be discussed in the section below). It is important that people living with ASC who access emergency services are encouraged to feel safe, have access to the information they need and have the presence and support of family and friends who understand their unique communication style, behaviour and emotions.

ASC affects 1 in 100 people and there are some 700,000 autistic adults and children in the United Kingdom [2]. ASC is one of the most common childhood-onset neurodevelopmental disorders with a male-to-female ratio of 3:1 to 5:1 prevalence of males to females across cited studies [12, 13]. This difference is attributed to the possibility that females may be more able to engage in social masking to "camouflage" their condition in order to "fit in" with societal norms though an element of under-reporting of girls may result in under-diagnosis.

ASCs are a form of neurodiversity with specific diagnostic criteria and a range of presentations. Some people maintain atypical eye contact such as staring at people for too long or avoiding eye contact, or intrusion into one's personal space by either standing too close to someone else, talking loudly or touching people inappropriately. Social naïveté and vulnerability to exploitation may be apparent as they may not always read into social situations and another person's agenda. A lack of social awareness may result in bluntness or lack of diplomacy and reduced empathy for the other person in social situations. Some people may experience difficulty understanding others' behaviour, motives and intentions; reading other people's facial expressions or vocal intonation. There may be a difficulty in conversational turn-taking or a tendency to dominate the conversation particularly relating to a fixated interest in a specialist subject. For some people, there may be an inability to make small talk or maintain a conversation and it may also be difficult for them to read between the lines or to pick up on hints. Preference for repetition and routine; need for sameness showing anxiety when faced with the possibility of change, preferring predictability. There may be a real attention to detail and a need for clarity and indeed, precision so avoiding ambiguity [12, 13].

According to the National Autistic Society, communication may be different in two ways first, concerning social communication and second, concerning social interaction. In social communication an autistic person may experience difficulty interpreting verbal and non-verbal language. In particular, hand gestures, posturing and signalling may be hard to interpret and the tone of voice that a person uses to express themselves may be hard to understand. Some autistic people may not be able to speak or may have limited speech whilst others may repeat what has been said (echolalia). Other autistic people may have very good language skills but struggle to understand conversational nuances such as sarcasm or tone of voice.

Utterances may be interpreted literally as the autistic person may not be able to conceptualise in an abstract way so additional time may be valuable as they process information.

Communication through social interaction can be affected by an inability to "read" other people and in recognising or understanding others' feelings and intentions. This inability to access and express their own emotions means that it can be hard to navigate the social world. As such, autistic people might seem insensitive, and tend to isolate, particularly when overloaded by other people. They may not seek comfort from other people and may appear to behave "strangely" or in a way thought to be socially inappropriate so it can be hard for them to form friendships.

It is important to note that, although an autistic "spectrum" is often quoted, this is not a linear entity. Each autistic person will have their own particular strengths and areas of challenge, creating their own unique, multi-faceted form of ASC. In order to help an autistic person to navigate the ED and access emergency healthcare, practitioners should gauge which factors (communication, social interaction, uncertainty, sensory processing for example) are likely to be more challenging and aim to make reasonable adjustments as appropriate.

The emergency environment provides many triggers which can heighten anxiety so it is not unusual for patients with ASC to display exaggerated responses. These can affect any of the senses, in many different ways. Sensations are processed by the body in an abnormal way which can cause either a painful or distressing experience (hypersensitive) or a lack of awareness of the sensation (hyposensitive). Not only can different sensations be perceived in different ways by different people, but they can vary for an individual also. Loud or sudden noises may be very painful to hear, a light touch might be very distressing and bright lights may be uncomfortable. These sensory messages have a huge impact on a person's ability to tolerate a visit to the ED where it is noisy, bright and hectic, with the added distress of blood pressure cuffs, saturation probes, stethoscopes, needles and so on.

The above behaviours and interpretations may prove overwhelming when faced with swift responses and complex activities carried out by practitioners during the emergency pathway. Consider a situation where a person with ASC and an altered Glasgow Coma Score is being prepared for a CT scan following a head injury which involves transfer to another location (imaging department) where they meet unfamiliar staff who give quite precise information over a speaker whilst the patient is scanned in a large, enclosed machine. Indeed, should an MRI scan be required for other conditions, this involves very loud intermittent noises which can unnerve even the most composed person. Think about the importance of family involvement and discuss what is the best way to prepare for these clinical procedures. Certainly, in the MRI context, it may be possible for someone close to accompany the patient if they feel able to cope with the excessive noise—patient sedation may also be considered.

6   Autistic Meltdown

Situations in which heightened sensory processing becomes exhausted may render the autistic person completely unable to cope and autistic meltdown may ensue. This may involve increased sensitivity to light, smell, heat, sound, taste and touch. In a BBC documentary, Sarinah, an autistic person, explained her meltdown as an attempt to "escape the chaos" inside her mind during what was an emotionally and physically painful experience [14]. It is important that the emergency practitioner separate their own feelings of anxiety about the patient's behaviour from the meltdown event. In Sarinah's words, "We're not giving a hard time, we're having a hard time". Her feelings of being defeated, judged and incompetent at not being able to get through what for neurotypical people may be an everyday encounter in a public place, are profound.

So, what can emergency practitioners do to support a person with ASC in the pre-hospital setting and emergency department, imaging department and on their journey through the system either to ward admission or discharge? Reasonable adjustments need to be in place to accommodate the needs of autistic people. Essentially, emergency practitioners should make every effort to make it as easy for people with autism to use emergency services as it is for people who do not have autism.

The signs of autistic meltdown tend to leak prior to the actual meltdown so during what is termed the 'rumble stage' the emergency practitioner should try to offer reassurance and create a calm environment, offering fidget toys, sunglasses, dimmed lighting or headphones to reduce the sensory overload. During an extreme response a range of behaviours may be displayed such as hand flapping, head hitting, kicking, pacing, rocking, hyperventilating, inability to communicate or total withdrawal into oneself. Emergency practitioners should not to try to break the cycle of behaviour but provide a private space away from public gaze which may help reduce mental overload for the patient.

It can be very helpful to the practitioner and ease the experience of the patient to find out whether your patient has sensory processing issues and how you may best be able to respond sensitively and effectively to them. A quiet room without machine beeps and raised voices can help, as can leaving more distressing parts of the assessment to the end of the examination. Engaging the help and advice of family and carers can make a huge difference and at the same time encourages them to feel that they are able to contribute as the person who is most familiar with the patient's needs. Distraction techniques might be useful for some although for others, who have been unfortunate enough to be in hospital multiple times, distraction may not be effective. Explanation and reassurance can go a long way, using appropriate communication techniques.

7   The Equality Act and Mandatory Training

The Equality Act (2010) [15] places a statutory obligation on all public sector organisations to provide reasonable adjustments to make changes in their approach or provision to ensure that services are accessible to disabled people as well as everybody else. Such adjustments may comprise easy-to-read information, prioritising patients or, giving more time to ensure the information given is understood.

Following the tragic death of Oliver McGowan, a light has been shone on the issue of how effective care and treatment is provided during the emergency pathway experience for people with ASC. Oliver was born prematurely, had mild autism, epilepsy and learning disabilities and in 2016 at Bristol emergency department he was administered olanzapine, an antipsychotic sedative, despite clear objection from his parents. This medication caused brain swelling among other symptoms and Oliver died in intensive care. This tragedy led to a national campaign urging healthcare staff to complete mandatory training in autism and learning disability awareness to "...ensure that every person who has autism and or intellectual disability receive the same medical care as everybody else in society, where their voices are heard and they are placed at the centre of their care" [16].

Resulting from the Oliver McGowan campaign mandatory training and a government-led consultation about provision of training and staff development around the issue of LD and autism, the UK Government 2019 consultation response set out their commitment to mandatory training in "Right to be heard". Funding was secured to develop and test a LD and autism training package for widespread rollout "The Oliver McGowan Mandatory Training in Learning Disabilities and Autism" with coproduction as the golden thread. The Interim Report (November 2021) showed a promising impact in that "74–95% of survey responders said that the training had made them more aware of the needs of people with a learning disability and autistic people" (p35) though further evaluations should reveal the full impact of the training.

8   Pain

LeDeR [5] reported that pain is an area often neglected when healthcare professionals are managing patients with LD. Possible reasons for this include difficulties in expressing pain for the individual with LD and challenges in assessment of pain by the clinician. LeDeR found that pain was not formally assessed as often in patients with LD, nor was it treated as vigorously. Often "pain thresholds" are described as being high or low, suggesting that painful stimuli are perceived in different ways by different individuals; a form of sensory processing disorder. Diagnostic overshadowing is also likely to play a large role. Pain and discomfort must be assessed and must be managed. A broken arm is a broken arm, whether the patient is able to describe the feeling or not, so should be treated in line with fracture management protocol. A pain score should be recorded, where possible. Symbols, signs, pictures or gestures can be used to identify localised pain. Pharmacological methods of pain relief should be used as they would be for any other patient, although consideration may need to be given to comorbid conditions, medication interactions and routes of administration. Consider whether or not less invasive measures such as intranasal opiates could be used instead of intravenous and also, if local anaesthetic gels such as LAT gel (lignocaine, adrenaline and tetracaine) could reduce the pain experience prior to wound management. Further, paracetamol suspension may be better tolerated than tablets. Do not forget non-pharmacological methods of pain relief such as splints, which may need some explanation or distraction to enable application.

9   Early Warning Scores

LeDeR also found that patients with LD were less likely to have an early warning score, such as NEWS2, calculated and, when it was calculated, it was less likely to be acted upon if found to be high. Early warning scores, although not perfect, have a valuable place in identifying unwell or deteriorating patients [17]. Issues can arise when patients have, or worse, are assumed to have, an abnormal score at baseline, and any subsequent abnormal scores are therefore presumed to be insignificant. This is another form of bias, akin to diagnostic overshadowing. Issues can also arise when a patient, due to underlying conditions, does not have an abnormal score, even when quite unwell. For example, some patients with neurological conditions may be unable to mount a pyrexia in response to infection, patients on betablockers may not be able to mount a tachycardia and patients with neuromuscular disorders may be unable to maintain an increased respiratory rate.

It is important, therefore, to look for other signs and symptoms of illness, beyond the early warning score. Having an idea of your patient's underlying condition may help you to understand more about how an early warning score may influence clinical assessment. It is also important, of course, to respond appropriately to high scores and not delay treatment either because of diagnostic uncertainty, or due to a fear of upsetting the patient or causing them distress. Treatments such as cannulation can be uncomfortable for any patient, with or without a LD, but discomfort can be reduced by the use of topical anaesthetic creams, good communication and, if needed, distraction. Not wanting to cause discomfort, whilst laudable, is not on its own a good enough reason to withhold potentially life-saving treatment, whether your patient has a LD or not.

On the theme of discomfort, some of the individual elements of early warning scores can be very uncomfortable for people with a LD, especially those with associated sensory processing disorder. This may be another factor that has led to the reduced frequency of scores being measured in this population. Again, appropriate care should be taken to explain, describe, distract and make the process as easy as possible for your patient. Consider a patient with a sensory processing disorder and communication difficulties, who does not understand what a "blood pressure" is. Think about how you might measure their blood pressure by perhaps showing them the cuff, allowing them to feel it and hold it. It may be helpful to demonstrate the technique to someone else first and also, to use symbols, pictures or signs. You may also need to think about how you might get them to hold their arm still throughout the measurement, especially as the increased tightness of the cuff could be distressing. Additionally, the noise of the machine may be disturbing so consider how distraction could be used by, e.g. giving them something else to hold or look at. In particular, it is always of comfort to have a friendly hand to hold.

10   The Mental Capacity Act

The Mental Capacity Act [18] was written, at least in part, to support people with a LD in making decisions about themselves and to give clarity to healthcare professionals making decisions for and with patients with reduced capacity. Unfortunately, it is often not well understood, including by many emergency practitioners, and often not appropriately followed [5]. The Act clearly states that everyone should be presumed to have capacity to make their own decisions, unless proven otherwise. All necessary steps must be taken to support a person in making decisions—practically, for ED staff, this means good communication, clear explanations, use of tools such as signs, symbols and easy-read documents, engaging the help of family and carers and taking extra time to ensure that the patient is able to understand, weigh up and retain the information. In emergency situations, this can be challenging and indeed not always possible. Capacity to make decisions varies with the nature and complexity of the decision and the situation. A person may be able to decide to accept a particular treatment one day, given the right circumstances, but not the next, if the circumstances are different. The Act tells us to always make every attempt possible to allow autonomous decision-making. Where those attempts are not successful, ED practitioners must ensure that decisions are made in the best interests of the patient. This can only happen if we take into account their individual needs and situation.

It is important to confirm if your patient has an Advanced Care Directive or if they have nominated someone to act on their behalf through a Lasting Power of Attorney. Independent mental capacity advocates can be a great resource for those without family or carers to support them through decision-making. Their role is to represent and support the person in relation to their "best interests". Individual Trusts will have their own referral pathways to access the Independent Mental Capacity Advocate (IMCA) system, often through the Safeguarding Team.

11   Resuscitation Decisions and Quality of Life

Assumptions should never be made about a person's quality of life—LD/autism or not. It is important to remember, when assessing a patient in the ED, that you may be seeing them at their lowest point, both physically and mentally. The combination of critical illness, difficulties with understanding and communication and distress caused by a change in environment, fear and differences in sensory processing can mean that the character in front of you is very different to that known and loved by friends and family.

Resuscitation and ceiling of care decisions should, of course, take into account quality of life, but information should be sought about this, and about other factors such as the patient's own wishes, from the patient and those who know them best. Consideration may need to be given as to whether or not your patient would be able to understand and tolerate particular procedures, but equally consideration must also be given regarding how clinicians can best help their patients (with or without LD/autism) to understand and tolerate those procedures and treatments which may be beneficial. Take, for example a patient with a LD who you think would benefit from non-invasive ventilation (NIV). Think about how you might explain what is going to happen and why it is important. Consider how you could mitigate against the discomfort and the noise and if it may be useful to encourage the patient to hold or touch the mask and to gradually increase the flow whilst they get used to it. Alternatively, a staff member might hold the mask on the patient's face, instead of using straps, at least to start. It may be possible to negotiate a short break after a period of treatment and in terms of distraction, it may be beneficial to provide a TV or tablet for them to watch. If they are very distressed. NIV may actually be a more appropriate option for them. Consider what the family and carers feel about the distress their loved one is facing and whether they might suggest anything to help and if a different treatment may be tolerated better. Indeed, high-flow nasal oxygen therapy might be less uncomfortable although less effective though intubation and ventilation might be considered if it is thought to be in the patient's best interests.

12   Hospital Passports

When family and carers are not able to pass on information then a hospital passport [19] can be helpful. Often in healthcare these are used for conveying lists of medications, allergies and past medical history. They have a role, also, in helping clinicians understand what matters to the patient such as how best to communicate with their patient, how to avoid unnecessary distress or whether or not distraction may be appropriate. Essentially, the hospital passport highlights areas that can make the hospital visit easier to tolerate for the patient and easier to navigate for the clinician. It may highlight particular sensory processing issues, e.g. knowing that taking a blood pressure is likely to be very distressing can help the ED practitioner to prepare for this. It may contain information about what the patient finds comforting perhaps indicating a favourite TV programme or if patient would benefit from having their favourite stuffed toy with them. The passport may indicate how best to communicate with the patient and the level of eye contact tolerated and, whether pictures or symbols would help? There may also be information about how best to help the patient settle if they do become distressed. When used properly, that is, properly completed and properly read, there may be a wealth of important information which could improve the assessment for both the patient and the practitioner.

13   Care Pathways

For some patients with significant learning disabilities and complex health needs, a care pathway can make a huge difference to their clinical management and their experience of healthcare. Ideally, these will be written by a team of multidisciplinary professionals with a combined knowledge of the health issues, communication challenges and difficulties with understanding that the individual faces, along with familiarity with the patient and their social situation. Family involvement can be very useful too. Care pathways should include plans for primary care involvement, when and how to transfer to hospital, how best to care for the patient in the ED environment and as an inpatient and any specific requirements for discharge planning. Care pathways, once written, then need to be easily accessible, easy to follow and updated when necessary. Flags and alerts on electronic patient records can help.

14   Family

Family members can be an incredibly valuable resource. They usually know their loved one best and are in a position to be able to describe how to communicate with them and how to maximise understanding and minimise distress. It is important, as healthcare professionals, to remember that we cannot know everything. Admitting this to our patient's family, and asking for their help, is not an admission of failure but acknowledgement of their role as carers and experts through lived experience. We need to trust the family and trust their judgement. We also need to do our best to gain their trust.

Bringing a loved one to the ED can be a very stressful experience for family members. They may be concerned for their welfare, worried that their concerns will not be taken seriously and wondering how best to make health professionals listen and understand. There may also have been previous traumatic experiences. Even planning and undertaking a visit to the hospital with a person with a LD can involve a great deal of time, energy and stress. It is important for ED staff to recognise this and to remain patient, attentive and understanding.

15   Soft Signs

Soft signs can be very helpful in identifying serious illnesses in patients with LD. These are things that families and carers will notice far more easily than healthcare professionals and it is vitally important that clinicians pay attention to their concerns. For example, Jack, a young man with Down syndrome, may appear more pale than usual when he is ill. He may be reluctant to get out of bed and may not want to eat his favourite food. He may not be interested in his favourite TV programme and his hands may be a little cool. Those factors, none of them specific to any particular illness, may be enough to let his family know that Jack is unwell. When there are so many challenges making recognition of serious illness more difficult in patients with LD, it is important to take note of soft signs, which may be unique to an individual and so not straightforward. There have been some attempts to formalise soft signs into systems for use in healthcare or even residential care settings [17, 20], making them another tool in the armoury for clinicians.

16   Learning Disability Nurses

LD nursing is a specialist area of nursing, for very good reason. Emergency Departments that are lucky enough to have access to an LD nurse should make the most of this, and their expertise, for both training purposes, case discussion and practical support and help with patients in the department.

17   Reasonable Adjustments

Reasonable adjustments [21] are required in law through the Equality Act, 2010 [22] which was written to protect people from discrimination. For ED staff this means making adjustments to usual practice to ensure that our patients with LD get the best care possible. Finding somewhere quiet for them to wait, making sure to communicate properly, taking time to listen and understand, providing easy-read information, for example are all adjustments that can make a huge difference to our patients. Some of these can be remembered with the TEACH mnemonic.

TEACH Mnemonic (REF)

T for Time – you may need to take extra time in your assessment

E for Environment – can you find somewhere quiet, with few distractions, reduced stimulation, perhaps with something familiar that can help your patient feel comfortable and safe?

A for Attitude – you need to keep an open mind, both about any potential diagnoses and about your patient's quality of life and ability to understand, given the right support.

C for Communication – find the best way to communicate with your patient. Speak slowly, clearly, avoid jargon. Consider use of signs or symbols. Give time for a response.

H for Help – what help does your patient need and how can you provide it? What help do you need in order to do this? Could you contact your Trust's Learning Disability nurse? Speak to family or carers? Access the Hospital Passport?

18   Staff Awareness

One of the first and biggest steps in improving outcomes for patients with LD is to ensure staff are aware of their needs and what matters most to them. Training is vitally important, as is ongoing access to resources and the opportunity to share best practice. A box of communication resources can be a helpful toolkit containing symbols, easy-read information, and guides to simple signing, for example. Another helpful toolkit can be a collection of sensory gadgets or toys to use for distraction or to calm an anxious patient.

Staff must be aware of the existence of hospital passports and care pathways, and know how to call a learning disability nurse. They must also be aware that they cannot know everything in every situation and that family and carers can be a valuable resource. It is also always worth remembering that family members can be very anxious and frustrated, wanting the best for their loved one and possibly remembering past negative experiences.

The ED Pledge for Patients with LD [23, 24] was formulated in the ED at Hull University Teaching Hospitals NHS Trust and has been shared at many other Trusts and departments. It is a collection of reasonable adjustments that all staff have promised to provide for their patients, to the best of their ability. They provide examples of good practice, which may be commonly overlooked in busy EDs.

Mencap led the *Treat Me Well* campaign [25] to improve awareness of LD amongst healthcare staff which involves training and cascading of information. The Oliver McGowan Mandatory Training in Learning Disability and Autism [26], named after a young autistic man who died after significant issues with his care, mentioned earlier in the chapter, is being rolled out at the time of writing and promises to address the need for training in this area.

19   Conclusion

Assessing and caring for a patient with a learning disability/autism in the ED can be a daunting prospect, but none of the challenges are insurmountable. The patient is likely to be far more nervous than the ED practitioner! There are many simple interventions we can consider which can improve the experience for our patients and help us to get the right clinical outcome for them, too. All of these are really just extensions of the good communication and patient-centred care we should already be providing, with reasonable adjustments made depending on the needs of our patients. Take time, consider your environment and attitude, pay attention to communication and use the people and resources [27] available to help you, so that you, in turn, can help your patient.

Learning Points
- Consider which barrier signs and tie signs you display during your interactions with people. How might you modify them when communicating with someone with LD and/or autism in the Emergency Department?

- Check whether your department has any resources such as PECS cards or Makaton symbols to aid communication with a person with LD. Could you learn some basic Makaton? Where could you find some easy-read discharge information?
- Consider five reasonable adjustments that you would make when caring for a patient with LD and/or autism in the emergency department.

References

1. MENCAP. Learning disabilities: Our definition. 2021. https://www.mencap.org.uk/learning-disability-explained/what-learning-disability
2. National Autistic Society. What is autism? 2021. https://www.autism.org.uk/advice-and-guidance/what-is-autism
3. MENCAP. How common is learning disability? 2021. https://www.mencap.org.uk/learning-disability-explained/research-and-statistics/how-common-learning-disability
4. University of Bristol. Confidential Inquiry into premature deaths of people with learning disabilities (CIPOLD) Final report. Bristol: University of Bristol; 2013. https://www.bristol.ac.uk/media-library/sites/cipold/migrated/documents/fullfinalreport.pdf
5. University of Bristol. The learning disabilities mortality review (LeDeR) Programme Annual Report (2019). Bristol: University of Bristol; 2019. http://www.bristol.ac.uk/sps/leder/
6. Hunt A. Sepsis: an overview of the signs, symptoms, diagnosis, treatment and pathophysiology. Emerg Nurse. 2019;27(5):32–41. https://doi.org/10.7748/en.2019.e1926.
7. Department for Work and Pensions/Office for Disability Issues. Guidance: accessible communication formats. UK Government Crown copyright, London. 2021. https://www.gov.uk/government/publications/inclusive-communication/accessible-communication-formats. Accessed 15 Mar 2021.
8. Makaton. About Makaton. 2021. https://makaton.org/TMC/AboutMakaton.aspx
9. Pyramid Educational Consultants. Picture exchange communication system. Brighton: (PECS) Pyramid Educational Consultants; 2021. https://pecs-unitedkingdom.com/pecs/
10. NHS England. Hearing care. 2021. https://www.england.nhs.uk/learning-disabilities/improving-health/eye-care-dental-care-and-hearing-checks/hearing-care/, https://www.england.nhs.uk/learning-disabilities/improving-health/eye-care-dental-care-and-hearing-checks/hearing-care/
11. National Development Team for Inclusion. Evaluation of the Oliver McGowan mandatory training in learning disabilities and autism: an interim report (November 2021). 2021.
12. NICE. Autism in adults: what is it? 2020. https://cks.nice.org.uk/topics/autism-in-adults/background-information/definition/
13. NICE Autism in adults: how common is it? 2020. https://cks.nice.org.uk/topics/autism-in-adults/background-information/prevalence
14. O'Donaghue S. BBC the social contributor. What are meltdowns? 2020. https://www.bbc.co.uk/programmes/articles/38f5MsC2mB5fnmCr5v77zDn/how-it-feels-to-have-an-autistic-meltdown-and-how-you-can-help. Accessed 29 Sept 2020.
15. GOV.UK. Equality Act 2010. Crown Copyright. Available at: "https://www.legislation.gov.uk/ukpga/2010/15/contents" Equality Act 2010 (legislation.gov.uk) [Accessed 11th March 2023.
16. Oliver's Campaign 2021. https://www.olivermcgowan.org/post/why-nhs-staff-should-receive-mandatory-training-in-autism-and-learning-disability
17. Gerry S, Bonnici T, Birks J, Kirtley S, Virdee PS, Watkinson PJ, Collins GS. Early warning scores for detecting deterioration in adult hospital patients: systematic review and critical appraisal of methodology. BMJ Open. 2020;369:m1501.

18. The Mental Capacity Act. Crown Copyright: London. 2005. https://www.legislation.gov.uk/ukpga/2005/9/contents
19. MENCAP. Hospital passports. 2021. https://www.mencap.org.uk/advice-and-support/health/health-guides
20. The Academic Health Science Network. Spotting the early 'soft signs' of deterioration and sepsis. 2020. https://www.ahsnnetwork.com/spotting-the-early-soft-signs-of-sepsis. Accessed 24 May 2020.
21. NHS England. Reasonable adjustments. 2021. https://www.england.nhs.uk/learning-disabilities/improving-health/reasonable-adjustments/
22. GOV.UK. Equality Act 2010: guidance. 27th February 2013 updated 16th June 2015. Crown Copyright: London; 2013. https://www.gov.uk/guidance/equality-act-2010-guidance
23. Hull University Teaching Hospitals NHS Trust. The emergency department pledge for people with learning disabilities. 2021. https://www.hey.nhs.uk/patients-and-visitors/children-learning-disabilities/the-emergency-department-pledge-for-people-with-learning-disabilities/
24. Makaton. Our pledge to people with learning disabilities: take the pledge be the change. 2019. https://youtube/xYbcZjdYbG0
25. MENCAP. Treat me well. 2021. https://www.mencap.org.uk/get-involved/campaign-mencap/treat-me-well, https://www.mencap.org.uk/get-involved/campaign-mencap/treat-me-well
26. Health Education England. The Oliver McGowan mandatory training in learning disability and autism. 2021. https://www.hee.nhs.uk/our-work/learning-disability/oliver-mcgowan-mandatory-training-learning-disability-autism
27. NICE. Autism spectrum disorder in adults: diagnosis and management. Clinical guideline [CG142]. 2021. Published: 27 June 2012. Last updated: 14 June 2021. https://www.nice.org.uk/guidance/cg142/chapter/Introduction

Paramedic

Joanne Mildenhall

1   Introduction

Paramedics and ambulance practitioners are often the healthcare professionals who have first contact with patients who are experiencing a psychiatric emergency, which may range from heightened anxiety through to self-harm, suicidal ideation or psychosis [1]. Such crises can be complex and influenced by a number of confounding psychosocial factors [2]. During such patient encounters, individuals can be greatly supported by a professional clinician-patient relationship that takes a calm and compassionate approach, whereby the person's concerns and needs are validated and psychological safety is promoted. Facilitating this may not always be easy, particularly if the practitioner feels inadequately prepared, lacks knowledge of psychological illness/management of conditions or feels under-confident in providing care in these situations [1, 3, 4].

Traditionally, the teaching of paramedicine has placed considerable focus on the clinical aspects of care and treatment for life-threatening medical emergencies which was representative of the core nature of ambulance response work. However, in more recent years, strategic policy and societal changes have influenced a shift in clinical practice, with a greater number of calls being received by the ambulance service from individuals requiring urgent healthcare needs – including for their mental health. Whilst paramedic educational programmes within the UK have progressed to incorporate aspects of urgent care within academic delivery, that pertaining to mental health crises and psychiatric emergencies is variable and, in some institutions, remains limited [1, 5]. Thus, it is unsurprising that some ambulance practitioners may feel ill-equipped both in knowledge and lack of experience, in

J. Mildenhall (✉)
Paramedic Psychological Health & Wellbeing Manager, College of Paramedics, Bridgwater, UK
e-mail: Joanne.Mildenhall@scas.nhs.uk

© The Author(s), under exclusive license to Springer Nature Switzerland AG 2023
T. Scott (ed.), *Mental Health: Intervention Skills for the Emergency Services*,
https://doi.org/10.1007/978-3-031-20347-3_3

making clinical decisions for patients with mental health needs. Arguably, this is more likely to be the case in crisis situations involving self-harm and/or suicidal intent which requires understanding and use of legislation, which can add further complexity [4, 6].

Research studies both in the UK and internationally advocated for improvements in the mental health education provided to pre- and post-registration paramedics, with recommendations for greater emphasis on patient assessment and management [3, 5, 7], a point which, perhaps, is of even more significance given the psychosocial and economic impact of the coronavirus pandemic upon people's mental wellbeing [8–10]. Although the effectiveness of mental health education upon practitioner confidence and patient care/outcomes has had limited exploration, a small pilot study undertaken by Green and Pound [11] researched the usefulness of a 2-week clinical placement with a mental health Trust. The authors found that undergraduate paramedic students rated the experience as positive as it provided them with greater understanding of mental ill-health and crisis, doing an assessment, the mental healthcare system and making referrals. Despite the small sample, the results indicated that such clinical experiences can be helpful in developing confident healthcare professionals.

Whilst discourse around mental health may be positively shifting within academic paramedicine, professional practice transformation, however, is yet to be robustly evidenced. Indeed, of the limited studies available, McCann et al. [5], identified that there was a tendency of ambulance practitioners to view such calls as a 'distraction' from 'the 'real' medical emergency work (such as resuscitation and incidents requiring critical intervention) that paramedics believe should be the primary focus of their work'. Perhaps a representative legacy attitude of emergency ambulance work, these views can hinder the ambulance professional in taking an open-minded and nonjudgemental approach to patients experiencing psychological ill-health and/or distress.

To give context, epidemiological data suggests that across the globe, a quarter of the population will experience mental ill-health at some point in their life [12]. Furthermore, the prevalence of mental illness within Britain is increasing, particularly when compared to pre-pandemic times [13]. Despite this, mental healthcare systems are frequently underfunded and inefficient due to unequitable public funding, austerity measures and limited/ restrictive provision within healthcare policy [14, 15]. Subsequently, the disparity in care between acute medicine and mental health is often evident in terms of reduced capability – including inaccessibility or protracted waiting times to access specialist psychological services, interventions and crisis care, particularly out-of-hours [16–18]. Consequently, people with mental health needs may find it difficult to access timely, psychological care. Thus, they are forced to try to manage their condition themselves, need to rely on family and/or friends to care for/support them (where available) or rely on alternative access to the health and social care system, such as via the ambulance service. Indeed, latest (pre-COVID) statistics indicated that 10–15% of all emergency ambulance calls received within England are of a psychiatric nature [19].

Whilst the distribution and patterns of these calls has not yet been mapped across the country, one retrospective analysis undertaken by North West Ambulance Service NHS Trust identified that over a 6-month period in 2019, of 46,869 emergency calls received, death from suicide was recorded in 124 incidents, with the most common method of suicide in the UK, hanging [20], being of highest prevalence [21]. Prior psychiatric ill health such as anxiety, self-harm or post-traumatic stress disorder and psychosocial issues such as substance abuse and relationship difficulties were notable in the history of those who had died, of which 18% had previously engaged with ambulance services for advice and care. The study recognised that two cohorts of patients were not included in this study: those who had attempted suicide but whom had been conveyed to the Emergency Department (ED) and those who had died following their hospital admission.

Although it is not yet known as to the exact impact the coronavirus pandemic has had upon ambulance calls for individuals experiencing psychological ill-health, we do know that associated psychosocial factors such as '...enforced social isolation', socio-economic hardship and 'significant loss of life' ([8], p.1) have brought additional challenges to our society and communities.

Early reports indicated that whilst the mental health trajectory for the majority of people was generally consistent and they were not adversely affected, analysis has identified trends in the development of emotional distress or crisis in those who have had no prior history of mental ill-health [22], and for those with a pre-existing mental health condition, some studies highlighted increasing numbers of people experiencing a deterioration in symptoms associated with anxiety and depression [10, 23]. Furthermore, the British Medical Association [8] raised awareness of the psychological impact of the pandemic upon healthcare workers, with many professionals, including ambulance staff, reporting heightened work-related stress and mental ill-health: an issue of considerable concern given the high prevalence of conditions such as post-traumatic stress disorder and suicide, prior to the pandemic [24, 25]. Thus, it is important to recognise that whilst ambulance clinicians may attend members of the public who require mental healthcare, they are just as (if not more) likely to experience psychological health needs of their own.

Whilst this chapter explores paramedicine perspectives on mental health in a general sense and details interventions in terms of approach, assessment and management, it is beyond the scope of this chapter to provide specific psychiatric presentations in detail nor explore in depth relevant mental health or capacity legislation.

2 Policy Guiding Practice

In terms of mental healthcare, a number of key policies and papers have been published that are relevant to paramedic practice. One of the most significant is the *Mental Health Crisis Care Concordat* [26], which is a shared statement agreement between agencies and services who care for people in mental health crisis. In recognising that individuals were often 'passed around' different agencies, with unacknowledged responsibility for care, the commitment laid out how organisations should work together to ensure that those experiencing mental distress are supported and receive the most appropriate and timely care to their needs. This includes police and ambulance services, mental health crisis teams and commissioners who fund and monitor services. Crisis Care Concordats should, essentially, improve the partnerships between such agencies, to ensure that individual's experiencing mental health crises are treated 'with the same urgency as physical health' needs and should be cared for by the health services, supported by the police where necessary. Where patients require further psychiatric assessment and support, they must be transported in a 'suitable vehicle'; often this will be an ambulance and conveyed to 'a health-based placed of safety rather than a police station' [26].

Subsequently, a report by the Care Quality Commission [27] set out to improve parity of esteem between physical and psychological health by improving mental health services, with a vision of standardising care across the country. A catalyst for change also came from NHS England [28] which took an integrated care approach in advocating for the development of psychiatric assessment and alternative care pathways (other than the ED) for those in crisis. Most recently, additional revenue was earmarked to fund specialist telephony triage by mental health professionals in ambulance control rooms, supplementary education for ambulance staff as well as funding for dedicated mental crisis response (such as street triage) in some areas [29]. The uncertain trajectory of the pandemic and rising demand for acute NHS services, however, has left the sustainability of new projects and long-term reform investment commitments in limbo [10].

In the wave of transformation of services and investment into mental health, reform of a key piece of legislation, the Mental Health Act 1983, is, at the time of publication, is also in progress. The Act provides the statutory framework for detaining and providing assessment, care and treatment for individuals experiencing severe psychological illness but who are unable to consent to their admission to hospital or for treatment. An independent review concluded that the Act is outdated and does not fit modern-day care provision, or our understanding and attitudes towards mental health which have evolved since its inception [30]. The recently published follow-up White Paper, *Reforming the Mental Health Act* lays out proposals for the legislative change, including a focus on choice and autonomy for patients, greater emphasis on respectful patient-centred, empowered care and treatment and using the powers in the least restrictive way. Furthermore, plans are underway which include tackling racial disparities experienced by individuals from minority ethnic groups who experience mental health crisis and to address '…underlying and systemtic racism that results in disproportionate detentions and use of force' mentioned by Sophie Corlett, Director of External Relations at Mind in the government Press Release *Landmark Reform of Mental Health Laws* [31].

3   Providing Care to Individuals with Mental Health Needs

Paramedics and ambulance practitioners are undoubtedly in a unique position. Arguably, they are well-placed to provide initial care for patients experiencing mental health needs and have some influence over the accessibility to local care pathways [1, 32, 33].

Patients' presentations and severity of mental ill-health may vary and fluctuate depending upon the nature of their illness, as well as a host of physiological, pharmacological and psychosocial factors such as perceived stressful life events, lack of sleep or medical conditions, for example, hypoglycaemia, brain tumours or Alzheimer's disease. For some, a mental health episode may be a one-off resulting in limited contact with the emergency or mental health services. For others, mental illness may be longer-term and involve more structured support and interventions within the community and hospital settings.

Due to the abstract nature of such presentations and associated emotional and behavioural responses, not knowing what to say or do to engage with patients who are mentally distressed can be a real worry for healthcare practitioners. Knowing how to gauge one's approach to an individual in crisis or distress can be difficult [1], particularly when a patient's emotions and behaviours are challenging, and may threaten our personal safety or that of themselves or bystanders. We may feel concerned that our interventions may make matters worse. Fortunately, there are some key things that we can do to approach and practically manage a mental health encounter in an impactful and positive way.

Providing care that treats an individual with dignity and compassion and is respectful of their needs, values and preferences is fundamental. Person-centred communication encourages and empowers patients in decision-making and therefore in co-creating personalised care. Through this process of rapport building and productive interactions, trust is promoted and is more likely to lead to a positive outcome for the patient. Co-creation of care is particularly helpful where a situation presents with complexities and where time is a factor. In this way, co-created care enables the person to be involved in determining what happens to them, thus alleviating any associated fear and anxiety. Establishing this relational dimension is essential for enabling patients to share in the responsibility for maintaining their own psychological health and wellbeing and ultimately quality of life [34]. One critical factor in developing a connection (rapport) between clinician and patient is the attitude and tone of the professional contact [1].

The disparity in professional education around psychological health and clinical science may unknowingly lead paramedics to view situations through a predominantly biomedical lens, whereby emphasis is placed upon the aetiology and pathophysiological underpinnings of an individual's presentation. This may inadvertently lead to biased attitudes on the part of the clinician, which subsequently could influence their approach and professional contact with a patient.

The importance of considering differential clinical diagnoses such as intoxication or head injury is paramount, but it can also be highly advantageous to take a broader, more holistic overview of the patient, their presentation and reason for reaching out to the ambulance service at that time [35]. In this way, practitioners may work in an integrative, personalised way to consider all aspects of a person rather than focusing entirely on symptoms and clinical diagnosis.

A psychosocial evaluation includes taking note of a person's living arrangements, family circumstances, availability of meaningful social support, lifestyle and habits, significant life events such as bereavement, chronic physical comorbidities and/or history of mental ill health. Gaining insight into past psychiatric history may be informative, but an overview of any key diagnoses is often enough in the pre-hospital setting to be able to then make professional decisions regarding further referrals and activate appropriate care pathways.

Whilst reflecting upon our own professional world views towards health and illness is vital in terms of understanding our relational approach, practice and care that we provide to patients, a greater sense of understanding may be gained from critical reflexion of our personal responses to the term 'mental health' and how this influences our interpretation of 'mental ill-health' and 'crisis'. As clinical professionals, this personalised consideration is fundamental to developing awareness of our preconceived thoughts, beliefs and attitudes that could, perhaps, inadvertently prejudice and stigmatise patients experiencing psychological health needs. Indeed, taking a nonjudgemental attitude is essential to providing dignified, person-centred care.

As noted, it is not the job of the paramedic to judge an individual's lifestyle choices or situation but rather to take a holistic and compassionate approach towards the person experiencing mental ill health and/or distress and to be considerate of the factors that may have led up to the point of contact. Building nonjudgemental, empathic rapport in this way is essential to good communication, collaboration and emotional regulation, thus de-escalating distress. This may be achieved through active and careful listening, open body language and asking open-ended questions, such as 'how are things for you at the moment?' or 'what's brought you to reach out to the ambulance service today?'.

Having only one or two people communicating with the patient at any time may reduce confusion and avoid the situation becoming overwhelming for the person. Similarly, if appropriate, and with the patient's agreement, reducing any distracting visual or audio stimulus such as the television, radio, social media, telephone calls and/or unhelpful bystanders may also help calm the environment. An individual who recalled a manic episode illustrates how sensory overload may be experienced:

> Everything is extremely bright and loud and everything inside my head is moving extremely fast. I'm irritated with everyone because no-one talks or does things as fast as I do. It's amazing but horrible at the same time...it's like I'm in my own amazing colourful world but everyone else is still stuck in the normal dull grey one.
> (Mind [36])

As the conversation progresses, it can be helpful to summarise and reflect back some of the things you have heard and to follow-up with closed or probing questions to gain insight into particular areas of concern and psychiatric symptoms. Examples include 'Do you feel that your mood has been quite low recently?' or 'I've noticed that you're taking x medication, are there any other medications that you've taken today?' or 'Are you in contact with your support worker?'. Careful questioning coupled with active listening and openness allow for psychological safety and trust to develop, thus engaging the patient and practitioner into meaningful communication [37, 38]. This allows for greater understanding and clarity of what has led to the current incident and how the patient is feeling and for collaborative discussion around onward care pathways.

When understanding has been gained of the events leading to the current situation and any relevant psychosocial and psychiatric history, it may be pertinent to assess mental capacity and undertake a brief mental health assessment. As detailed in the Joint Royal Colleges Ambulance Liaison Committee clinical guidelines [39], a brief mental health assessment includes observations such as the individual's appearance, behaviours, the rapport they have with others, their thoughts, mood, emotions and the insight that they have into their own reality.

An alternative is the 'ABCDE' model of assessment:

A Appearance - do they appear neglected, dishevelled or inappropriately dressed for the weather/environment?

B Behaviour - are they disinhibited, impulsive, bizarre, aggressive, unpredictable or withdrawn?

C Communication - is their speech incoherent, rapid, disconnected, confused or limited/uncommunicative?

D Ideation - note any beliefs, delusions, preoccupied, perception, hallucinations and irrational thought processes.

E Emotion - is the person excitable, euphoric, suspicious, sad, inappropriate to situation, rapidly changing (labile) or distressed?

(Doy et al. [37]

Where possible, it can sometimes help to encourage the individual to focus and talk through practical solutions themselves as this can be empowering and enable them to see the choices that they have and the outcomes available. Indeed, in this way, people can be enabled, within reason, to self-manage their condition/symptoms. Providing appropriate information at a pace and in a way that the person can understand, can help them to make informed choices and is respectful of their autonomy.

---

4   Patients Experiencing Challenging Behavioural and Emotional Crisis

Engaging with patients who are relatively calm, co-operative and have the focused ability to think things through rationally is one thing; however, sometimes this is not the case. Patients who are highly agitated, experiencing acute psychosis and/or experiencing heightened emotions such as anger or distress for example may present in ways that may be challenging for a healthcare professional and, sometimes, not conducive to a safe approach. In these instances, paramedics and ambulance personnel should undertake an assessment of risk to themselves, the patient and others [37] and follow local guidance for gaining further support which may include requesting police assistance, critical care and/or mental health crisis physicians.

Although agitation can be a common presentation of many psychiatric illnesses including schizophrenia, bipolar disorder and dementia, often underlying such distress are heightened levels of fear, inner anger/tension, anxiety, hypervigilance of one's surroundings/people and feeling restless or out-of-control [40]. An intense, unpredictable, emotional and behavioural response may also occur when usual coping strategies are insufficient to manage stressful situations, and an individual becomes overwhelmed and feels unable to cope. In other cases, agitation could be relatable to side effects from psychiatric medications or poor medicine compliance [41]. Both behavioural and emotional responses may be exacerbated by alcohol consumption and/or cannabis or other drugs use [42]. Furthermore, high stimulus environments with loud noises, numerous people, sirens, etc. will likely heighten the person's feeling of being overwhelmed to the point of sensory overload.

Whilst de-escalation through non-pharmacological means such as talking someone down, offering reassurance and building rapport are preferable, the situation may rarely be such that antipsychotics (e.g. olanzapine), benzodiazepines (e.g. lorazepam, midazolam) or other pharmacological sedatives are required for the safe management of the patient. Physical restraint may be necessary but must always be a last resort where it is needed and by the least restrictive method, to keep the patient and others safe from harm. In these instances, hospital admission to an ED is the usual outcome, where nonpsychiatric aetiology (such as head injury, infection, metabolic disorders, seizures, stroke, drug use or gestational/post-natal related disorders) can be excluded [42, 43]. Where possible, paramedics should attempt to gain a set of vital signs including oxygen saturations, blood pressure, temperature, blood glucose reading and level of consciousness [37, 39]. Abnormal measurements may be indicative of medical rather than psychiatric differential diagnoses. However, scoping the relevant past medical, pharmacological, psychiatric and psychosocial history will also be key.

5   Interventions for Mental Health Illness and Crisis

For many individuals, referral for mental health support from community mental health teams (CMHT) comprised of psychiatric nurses, social workers, psychiatrists, etc. is appropriate and sufficient. For those experiencing acute, severe illness, it may be necessary to draw upon the Mental Health Act (MHA, 1983) to provide further statutory guidance. In England and Wales, this legislative framework allows for detainment and urgent assessment and treatment (usually in-hospital) of individuals who are experiencing a mental health disorder and are at risk of serious harm to themselves and/or others. Depending upon which section of the Act is to be used, detention for involuntary hospital admission may be initiated by a police officer (e.g. in the case of s135 or s136), or an application for detention may be made by an Approved Mental Health Professional (AMHP) upon the basis of recommendations from two suitably qualified doctors. In these instances, ambulance practitioner's may be required to instigate the process by initiating a professional conversation with the AMHP and/or to transport individuals who have been detained ('sectioned') under the MHA (1983).

Box 1 Sections of the Mental Health Act (1983) most relevant to the ambulance sector

Section of the act	
Section 2	Admission for assessment (up to 28 days)
Section 3	Admission for treatment (up to 6 months)
Section 4	Admission for assessment in cases of emergency
Section 36	Remand to hospital for treatment
Section 48	Removal to hospital of unsentenced prisoners
Section 135	Police power (with a warrant) to detain and remove a person believed to be mentally disordered, from their home to a place of safety for assessment
Section 136	Police power (without a warrant) to detain a person in a public place who is believed to be mentally disordered and in need of immediate care/control, and remove to, or keep at, a place of safety for assessment

In other situations, paramedics may be called to attend individuals who express suicidal ideation, thoughts of serious self-harm or have, indeed, attempted the act. In many instances, by the arrival of the ambulance service, the patient has moved forwards in their thinking and is often open to assessment and further onward care. However, for others, they may well be intent on ending their own life, or they may express their wish to do so in the imminent future. In these cases, it is important to establish the 'likely physical risk, and the person's emotional and mental state, in an atmosphere of respect and understanding' ([44], p.54). Risk should include consideration of the effects of the self-injurious act (such as overdose or substance misuse) that has occurred and likely effects if no treatment is given. Contacting the national poisons information database to obtain specific information as to these effects is good practice and can help the practitioner to make a decision concerning the most suitable treatment/care plan and the clinical advice that they should provide to the patient.

The assessment and management of suicidal risk is complex, and its measurement is an area of contention within the psychiatric world. To date, there is no universally accepted evidence-based framework for adequately measuring or predicting this risk. Of the scales that are in use, research has now identified that they are not helpful and not good predictors of that risk and therefore insufficient in determining a particular care pathway or treatment that would be of benefit to an individual [20, 45]. For some time, the 'IPAP' risk assessment model was utilised within UK paramedic clinical guidelines, but, in the latest publication, this is now removed [39]. Rather, emphasis is placed upon a structured, person-centred approach to assessing current social and psychological health needs that identifies risk factors and mediators, which is best for informing the onward management of the patient's care [38].

When working with a person who has expressed suicidal ideation or thoughts of self-harm, building relationship is essential to encourage engagement and for collaborative decision-making. Ambulance practitioners are encouraged to include the individual in discussions around involving their family, carers or significant others [46]. Encouraging hope and thoughts for a better future can sometimes help a person to psychologically move forwards beyond the dark place which they occupy.

Shared decision-making is particularly important in complex cases such as situations where life may be at risk. This includes incidents where patients have self-harmed and are refusing assessment or treatment and decision-making around a person's mental capacity at that time and any issues around consent [44]. In these circumstances, the sharing of 'need to know' information between different agencies or with senior clinicians is appropriate and considered good practice [47]. This may include personal details, information about their current presentation and risk factors such as self-neglect and self-harm. It may be that the individual has a mental health crisis plan in place that has been agreed by the patient and their mental health team and may aid paramedics in their decision-making around what to do next. Documenting the clinical and mental assessments and decisions undertaken is essential.

6   Integrated Care Interventions, Pathways and Referrals

It is understandable that given the complexities of mental ill-health, paramedics may feel unease at discharging patients on scene, and as noted above, best practice in complex cases advocates shared decision-making and advice from experts within the field. However, it is notable that accessing appropriate referral pathways for specialist community mental health services can be very difficult [6], leaving little option but to convey the patient to an ED. This is often not the preferred place of care or the most appropriate location for those experiencing an episode of mental ill health [4, 48, 49] and may also lead to clinical assessments being duplicated as well as exacerbated wait times to access specialist help (NHS England, 2016).

As previously discussed, national policy developments in the NHS Long Term Plan proposed recommendations for enhancing crisis care and focus on the use of alternative care pathways to allow for patients to receive timely care and treatment in the community [19, 29]. Integrated care systems (ICS) or sustainability and transformation partnerships (STP's) formulated urgent care networks to promote collaborative working and funding of services. This includes the '111' urgent healthcare telephone service which is advocated to become the single point of access for people who reach out for help with mental ill health. The aim of both ICS and STP's is to safely reduce the conveyance of patients to the ED and to streamline urgent care services [19]. However, the pathways and outcomes in relation to mental health are yet to be analysed. Interventions that have seemingly been popular amongst ambulance staff and patient's alike are the development of 'hear and treat' pathways, such as mental health triage available in ambulance control rooms, and 'see and treat' street triage cars, typically staffed by a mental health practitioner and a paramedic, who provide an emergency response to calls from patients experiencing mental ill-health, crisis or distress.

O'Hara et al. [50] undertook pilot research within Yorkshire Ambulance Service NHS Trust to evaluate the usefulness of mental health nurses in triaging calls in the Emergency Operations Centre (EOC). Through a mixed-method evaluation and semi-structured interviews, the authors found that clinical staff viewed the introduction of specialist triage by mental health nurses as positive to service delivery by enhancing the patient care journey. Furthermore, emergency ambulance practitioners felt that the mental health nurses brought them a greater awareness of mental health issues and perceived that the nurses' professional connections within the mental health field was invaluable in gaining the most appropriate care for patients. However, these findings were based on a very limited sample of only 12 staff: 2 of whom were paramedics, and 3 were mental health nurses; thus, the results are limited in terms of representativeness and transferability. This aspect of the study also did not take account of the personal experiences of patients, relatives or carers.

Quantitative findings from incident call data on the other hand showed that mental health triage resulted in a greater number of 'hear and treat' calls, with a reduction in the number of ambulances dispatched and the total numbers of patients who were conveyed to hospital. Whilst this was a positive outcome, it was acknowledged that challenges presented due to the quick instigation of the pilot study, which affected the promotion of the service to all clinical staff.

In another pilot study, NHS Improvement [51] commissioned six mental health nurses to triage calls and provide a 'hear and treat' service to patients with complex mental health needs in London as part of an integrated care service. Key interventions include screening calls, referring patients to community mental health teams, providing training and supervision for staff, supporting ambulance crews with specialist advice and providing expert guidance on complex cases involving, for example, the Mental Health Act or Mental Capacity Act. Following a 1-month study period, the findings showed that, on average, the nurses dealt with 38 calls per 24-h period. The service '…improved London Ambulance Service NHS Trust staff confidence and ability to manage patients in mental health crisis, reduced avoidable ambulance dispatches and reduced avoidable journeys to the Emergency Department' ([51, 52], p. 1). Over a 1-year period, the service accounted for 954 cases via hear and treat. A key learning from this process was the need for effective communication and working relationships with partner organisations with a shared understanding for each other's roles and capabilities.

Whilst challenges were noted in the implementation and running of the above projects, overall, there were many positive benefits in terms of enhanced service delivery and transformation in providing timely specialist patient care in a telephonic way and reducing the demand upon physical ambulance response. In addition, the results indicated that multidisciplinary relationships were enriched with greater understanding of the contributions each professional could make to an individual's care and wellbeing through collaborative planning and decision-making. One area that still needs further investigation in relation to integrated care systems such as mental health practitioners triaging calls is the impact of this service upon individuals who have complex needs and are high-intensity users of the ambulance service, as well as other patient groups such as those with comorbidities of substance misuse and long-term medical conditions. These patients may well benefit from a consistent approach and may have an agreed care plan in place with direct links to their community team [53]. It was proposed that ambulance clinicians and mental health nurses will be able to access the National Record Locator Service, to ascertain an individual's agreed crisis plan, therefore aiding clinical decision-making around providing follow-up care via community pathways [54]. Indeed, a successful interoperability pilot programme was undertaken within London Ambulance Service between 2018–2020 [55].

Whilst these systems utilise the mental health professional's expertise, in the future it is wholly possible that paramedics may become skilled as specialist or advanced practitioners in mental health, particularly given the national shortage of workers within this field and the increasing rise in patient numbers. However, at the time of writing, this is not currently a formal professional or educational pathway available to paramedics.

Other models of alternative care which paramedics can refer a patient to are also coming to fruition. In some areas of the country, we have seen the development and opening of 'crisis cafes', 'crisis sanctuaries' and 'safe havens' for people to drop in and seek support from mental health practitioners when they are feeling emotionally distressed or in crisis. In Oxfordshire, telepsychiatry, one of the first services of its kind in the UK is currently being trialled, for which patients presenting with mental ill health at outreach hospitals can be triaged via video conferencing from the county's major acute hospital. In this way, complex cases may be quickly reviewed and followed up with appointments via electronic medium as required [56].

Another intervention, social prescribing, is a relatively new concept which is not yet available in all areas of the country. This method takes a holistic, psychosocial approach to supporting people with their health and wellbeing and can initially be accessed through a person's general practitioner, social worker, etc. Through encouragement from a link worker, individuals are connected with non-clinical services, community groups and statutory services which provide both emotional and practical support. The aim is to empower people to manage their symptoms, reduce isolation and loneliness and get help with debt, housing and employment, as well as lifestyle and nutritional advice. Thus, in turn these interventions may improve psychosocial wellbeing and, subsequently, mental health [57].

7   Conclusion

Providing care to patients who are experiencing psychological health needs is commonplace within contemporary paramedic practice. This can provide rewarding opportunity for ambulance practitioners to deliver person-centred care and to utilise their clinical and professional knowledge to formulate appropriate onward referral. However, limited education and experience on the part of the professional can make calls of this nature personally challenging, and there is a real need to enhance academic provision around mental health/illness to strengthen clinical competence and confidence. Nevertheless, collaborative working alongside psychiatric experts within integrated care systems cannot be underestimated in terms of providing quality patient care and appropriate referral. With the advent of new, innovative practices within the field of psychiatry including telemedicine, telephone triage, community hubs and social prescribing, patients, and paramedics alike, may see the range of supportive services widen to meet both psychological and psychosocial needs.

Learning Points
- Outline the section of mental health legislation which impacts on patients in the pre-hospital setting.
- Consider your own approach to people presenting with a mental health condition. What are your immediate concerns?
- Outline recently introduced partnership arrangements to support people with mental health needs in the pre-hospital setting.

References

1. Keefe B, Carolan K, Wint AJ, Goudreau M, Cluett S, Lezzoni LI. Behavioral health emergencies encountered by community paramedics: lessons from the field and opportunities for skills advancement. J Behav Health Serv Res. 2020;47:365–76.
2. Ross L, Jennings P, Williams B. Psychosocial support issues affecting older patients: a cross-sectional paramedic perspective, inquiry. J Med Care Org Provision Financing. 2017;54
3. Berry M. College of Paramedics' Evidence into Mental Health Care and Policing. J Param Pract. 2014;6(10):539–40.
4. Morrison-Rees S, Whitfield R, Evans S, Snooks HA. Investigating the volume of mental health emergency calls in the Welsh Ambulance Service Trust (WAST) and developing a pre-hospital mental health model of care for application and testing. Emerg Med J. 2015;32(5):e3. https://doi.org/10.1136/emermed-2015-204880.8.
5. McCann TV, Savic M, Ferguson N, Bosely E, Smith K, Roberts L et al (2018) Paramedics' perceptions of their scope of practice in caring for patients with non-medical emergency-related mental health and/or alcohol and other drug problems: a qualitative study, PLoS One, 13, 12, e0208391. https://journals.plos.org/plosone/article?id=10.1371/journal.pone.0208391. Accessed 1 Apr 2021.
6. Zayed MG, Williams V, Glendenning AC, Bulger JK, Hewes T, Porter A, Snooks H, John A. Care pathways for patients presenting to emergency ambulance services with self-harm: national survey. Emerg Med J. 2020;37:752–5.
7. Uddin T, Saadi A, Fisher M, Cross S, Attoe C. Simulation Training for Police and Ambulance Services to Improve Mental Health Practice. J Mental Health Training Educ Pract. 2020;15(5):303–14.
8. British Medical Association. The impact of COVID-19 on mental health in England: supporting services to go beyond parity of esteem. 2020. Available at: https://www.bma.org.uk/media/2750/bma-the-impact-of-covid-19-on-mental-health-in-england.pdf. Accessed 20 Jan 2022.
9. Mind. Coronavirus: the consequences for mental health. 2021. Available at: https://www.mind.org.uk/media/8962/the-consequences-of-coronavirus-for-mental-healthfinal-report.pdf. Accessed 4 Jan 2022.
10. Thorlby R, Tallack C, Finch D, Idriss O, Rocks S, Kraindler J, Shembavnekar N, Alderwick H. The health foundation – spending review 2020: priorities for the NHS, social care and the nation's health. 2020. Available at: https://www.health.org.uk/publications/long-reads/spending-review-2020. Accessed 21 Sept 2021.
11. Green A, Pound A. Undergraduate paramedics' understanding of mental health insight placements. J Param Pract. 2020. Available at: https://www.paramedicpractice.com/features/article/undergraduate-paramedics-understanding-of-mental-health-insight-placements. Accessed 16 Sept 2021.
12. World Health Organization. Depression and other common mental disorders: global health estimates. Geneva: World Health Organization; 2017.
13. Office for National Statistics. Coronavirus and depression in adults, Great Britain: January to March 2021. 2021. Available at: https://www.ons.gov.uk/peoplepopulationandcommunity/wellbeing/articles/coronavirusanddepressioninadultsgreatbritain/januarytomarch2021. Accessed 11 Oct 2021.
14. Mind. Mind responds to UK government's spring budget. 2021. Available at: https://www.mind.org.uk/news-campaigns/news/mind-responds-to-uk-governments-spring-budget/. Accessed 11 Oct 2021.
15. The Kings Fund. Funding and staffing of NHS mental health providers: still waiting for parity. 2018. Available at: https://www.kingsfund.org.uk/publications/funding-staffing-mental-health-providers. Accessed 19 Sept 2021.

16. Mental Health Today. Referrals for mental health services surge across Great Britain. 2021. Available at: https://www.mentalhealthtoday.co.uk/news/government-policy/referrals-for-mental-health-services-surge-across-great-britain. Accessed 10 Oct 2021.

17. Pretner C, Lincoln AK. Emergency Medical Services and 'Psych Calls': Examining the Work of Urban EMS Providers. Am J Orthopsychiat. 2015;85(6):612–9.

18. Rimmer A Mental health: staff shortages are causing distressingly long waits for treatment, college warns, Br Med J. 2021. Available at: https://doi.org/10.1136/bmj.n2439. Accessed 20 Jan 2022.

19. NHS England and NHS Improvement. Planning to safely reduce avoidable conveyance: ambulance improvement project. 2019. Available at: https://www.england.nhs.uk/wp-content/uploads/2019/09/planning-to-safetly-reduce-avoidable-conveyance-v4.0.pdf. Accessed 1st Apr 2021.

20. Appleby L, Kapur N, Shaw J, et al. National confidential inquiry into suicide and safety in mental health, annual report, England, Northern Ireland, Scotland and Wales 2019. Manchester: University of Manchester; 2019. https://www.research.manchester.ac.uk/portal/en/projects/national-confidential-inquiry-into-suicide-and-safety-in-mental-health(788f9475-cadb-4697-bb82-817638044b7b).html. Accessed 20 Jan 2022.

21. Hayden C, Moat C, Newbury-Birch D. Analysing ambulance data to ascertain the prevalence and demographics of individuals who have died by suicide. Emerg Nurs. 2020. https://doi.org/10.7748/en.2020.e2035. Accessed 2 Apr 2021.

22. Mental Health Foundation. Nine-Month Study Reveals Pandemic's Worsening Emotional Impacts on UK Adults. 2021. Available at: https://www.mentalhealth.org.uk/news/nine-month-study-reveals-pandemics-worsening-emotional-impacts-uk-adults. Accessed 20 Sept 2021.

23. Pierce M, McManus S, Hope H, Hotopf M, Ford T, Hatch S, John A, Kontopantelis E, Webb RT, Wessely S, Abel K. Different mental health responses to the COVID-19 pandemic: latent class trajectory analysis using longitudinal UK data. Lancet. 2021. Available at: https://papers.ssrn.com/sol3/papers.cfm?abstract_id=3784647. Accessed 20 Sept 2021.

24. Hird K, Bell F, Mars B, James C, Gunnell D. OP6 an investigation into suicide amongst ambulance staff. Emerg Med J. 2019. Available at: https://emj.bmj.com/content/36/1/e3.1. Accessed 11 Oct 2021.

25. Mars B, Hird K, Bell F, James C, Gunnell J. Suicide among ambulance service staff: a review of coroner and employment records. Br Param J. 2020;4(4):10–5.

26. HM Government. Mental health crisis care concordat: improving outcomes for people experiencing mental health crisis. 2014. Available at: https://assets.publishing.service.gov.uk/government/uploads/system/uploads/attachment_data/file/281242/36353_Mental_Health_Crisis_accessible.pdf. Accessed 26 Jan 2021.

27. Care Quality Commission. Right here, right now: people's experiences of help, care and support during a mental health crisis. 2015. Available at: https://www.cqc.org.uk/sites/default/files/20150630_righthere_mhcrisiscare_full.pdf. Accessed 20 Jan 2022.

28. NHS England. Transforming urgent and emergency care services in England. Safer, faster, better: good practice in delivering urgent and emergency care. A guide for local health and social care communities. Version number: 28 FINAL. 2015. https://www.england.nhs.uk/wp-content/uploads/2015/06/trans-uec.pdf. Accessed 31 Mar 2022.

29. NHS. The NHS Long Term Plan. 2019. Available at: https://www.longtermplan.nhs.uk/wp-content/uploads/2019/08/nhs-long-term-plan-version-1.2.pdf. Accessed 1 April 2021.

30. Department of Health & Social Care. Modernising the mental health act: increasing choice, reducing compulsion – final report of the independent review of the mental health act 1983. 2018. Available at: https://assets.publishing.service.gov.uk/government/uploads/system/uploads/attachment_data/file/778897/Modernising_the_Mental_Health_Act_-_increasing_choice__reducing_compulsion.pdf. Accessed 2 Apr 2021.

31. Department of Health & Social Care. Landmark reform of mental health laws. 2021. Available at: https://www.gov.uk/government/news/landmark-reform-of-mental-health-laws. Accessed 26 Jan 2022.

32. College of Paramedics. Paramedic Career Framework. 3rd ed. Bridgewater: College of Paramedics; 2016. Available at: https://www.collegeofparamedics.co.uk/COP/Professional_development/interactive_career_framework/COP/ProfessionalDevelopment/Interactive_Career_Framework.aspx?hkey=5058228a-13ef-4d38-a7b0-255e6263c9f7. Accessed 20 Jan 2022.

33. Shaban R. Paramedics clinical judgement and mental health assessments in emergency contexts: research, practice and tools of the trade. J Emerg Primary Health Care. 2006;4:2. Available at: https://ajp.paramedics.org/index.php/ajp/article/view/369/369. Accessed 12 Oct 2021.

34. NHS England. Involving People in their Own Care. 2021. Available at: https://www.england.nhs.uk/ourwork/patient-participation/. Accessed 13 Sept 2021.

35. Ford-Jones PC, Chaufan C. A critical analysis of debates around mental health calls in the prehospital setting. Inquiry. 2017; https://doi.org/10.1177/0046958017704608. Available at: https://www.ncbi.nlm.nih.gov/pmc/articles/PMC5798668/. Accessed 3 Apr 2021.

36. Mind. Hypomania and mania. 2021. Available at: https://www.mind.org.uk/information-support/types-of-mental-health-problems/hypomania-and-mania/about-hypomania-and-mania/. Accessed 12 Oct 2021.

37. Doy R, Blowers EJ, Sutton E. 16 mental health. Emerg Med J. 2006;23(4):304–12.

38. National Collaborating Centre for Mental Health. Self-harm and suicide prevention competence framework: adults and older adults. 2018. Available at: https://www.ucl.ac.uk/pals/sites/pals/files/self-harm_and_suicide_prevention_competence_framework_-_adults_and_older_adults_8th_oct_18.pdf. Accessed 10 Apr 2021.

39. Joint Royal Colleges Ambulance Liaison Committee, Association of Ambulance Chief Executives. JRCALC Clinical Guidelines. Cited from: JRCALC Plus (2017). Bridgewater: Class Publishing Ltd; 2021. Accessed 3 April 2021.

40. Roberts J, Canales AG, Blanthorn-Hazell S, Boldeanu AC, Judge D. Characterising the experience of agitation in patients with bipolar disorder and schizophrenia. BMC Psychiatry. 2018;18:104. Available at: https://bmcpsychiatry.biomedcentral.com/articles/10.1186/s12888-018-1673-3. Accessed 4 April 2021.

41. Poyurovsky M. Acute Antipsychotic-induced akathisia revisited. Br J Psychiat. 2010;196(2):89–91.

42. San L, Marksteiner J, Zwanzger P, Figuero MA, Romero FT, Kyropoulos G, Peixoto AB, Chirita R, Boldeanu A. Stage of acute agitation at psychiatric emergencies in Europe: the STAGE study. Clin Pract Epidemiol Mental Health. 2016;12:75–86.

43. Zeller SL, Citrome L. Managing agitation associated with schizophrenia and bipolar disorder in the emergency setting. West J Emerg Med. 2016;17(2):165–72. https://doi.org/10.5811/westjem.2015.12.28763. Epub 2016 Mar 2

44. The British Psychological Society/The Royal College of Psychiatrists. Self-harm. The short-term physical and psychological management and secondary prevention of self-harm in primary and secondary care. National Clinical Practice Guideline Number 16. 2004. p. 54. https://www.nice.org.uk/guidance/cg16/evidence/full-guideline-189936541. Accessed 31 Mar 2022.

45. Large M, Ryan C, Carter G, Kapur N. Can we usefully stratify patients according to suicide risk? Br Med J. 2017;359:j4627.

46. Health Education England. Paramedic specialist in primary and urgent care core capabilities framework. 2018. https://www.hee.nhs.uk/sites/default/files/documents/Paramedic%20Specialist%20in%20Primary%20and%20Urgent%20Care%20Core%20Capabilities%20Framework.pdf. Accessed 31 Mar 2022.

47. Mind. Confidentiality and information sharing. For carers, friends and relatives. 2016. https://www.mindcharity.co.uk/wp-content/uploads/2015/10/Confidentiality-Information-Sharing.pdf. Accessed 31 Mar 2022.

48. Heyland M, Johnson M. Evaluating an alternative to the emergency department for adults in mental health crisis. Issues Mental Health Nurs. 2017;38(7):557–61.

49. Mind. Listening to experience: an independent inquiry into acute and crisis mental health-care. 2011. Available at: www.mind. org.uk/media/211306/listening_to_experience_web.pdf. Accessed 1st Apr 2021.

50. O'Hara R, Irving A, Johnson M and Harris A. Service Evaluation of a Triage Pilot Intervention for Ambulance Service patients with Mental Health Problems. 2016. Available at: https://www.sheffield.ac.uk/polopoly_fs/1.647212!/file/YAS_Mental_Health_Triage_Report.pdf. Accessed 3 Apr 2021.

51. NHS Improvement. Introducing mental health nurses to the emergency operations centre at the London Ambulance Service. 2016. Available at: https://improvement.nhs.uk/documents/330/Case_study_-_LAS_mental_health.pdf. Accessed 2 Apr 2021.

52. London Ambulance Service NHS Trust. Mental Health Care. 2021. Available at: https://www.londonambulance.nhs.uk/calling-us/mental-health-care/. Accessed 2 April 2021.

53. Royal College of Emergency Medicine. Mental Health in emergency departments: a toolkit for improving care. 2019. Available at: https://www.rcem.ac.uk/docs/RCEM%20Guidance/Mental%20Health%20Toolkit%202019%20-%20Final%20.pdf. Accessed 2 Apr 2021].

54. NHS Digital. Mental health crisis plan access for ambulance staff to go live. 2019. Available at: https://digital.nhs.uk/news/2019/mental-health-crisis-plan-access-for-ambulance-staff-to-go-live. Accessed 20 Jan 2022.

55. Calpin J. National record locator programme; a feature by NHS Digital. Health Tech Newspaper. 2020. Available at: https://htn.co.uk/2020/11/16/national-record-locator-programme-a-feature-by-nhs-digital/. Accessed 20 Jan 2022.

56. The Health Foundation. Introducing telepsychiatry into routine practice in an emergency department psychiatric service. Available at: https://www.health.org.uk/improvement-projects/introducing-telepsychiatry-into-routine-practice-in-an-emergency-department. Accessed 2 Apr 2021.

57. Office for Health Improvement & Disparities. Social prescribing: applying all our health. 2022. Available at: https://www.gov.uk/government/publications/social-prescribing-applying-all-our-health/social-prescribing-applying-all-our-health. Accessed 4 Jan 2023.

Police Custody Officer

Ruth McGrath

1   Introduction

A fundamental and undisputed purpose of the UK police service since its inception is the protection of life [1]. This concept covers a broad range of incidents dealt with on a daily basis across the police service, by police officers, volunteers such as special constables and those in public facing support roles, including the Police Community Support Officer (PCSO), enquiry desk staff and detention officers. One increasingly expanding demand concerns the protection of vulnerable persons, some of whom may experience mental ill-health.

The term mental ill-health is broadly used in this chapter to encompass those who are vulnerable because they are experiencing mental ill-health or with multiple needs resulting from their mental health. Terminology has adjusted over time, including 'mental health disorder' [2, 3], 'mentally vulnerable' [4, 5], 'mental health condition' [5, 6], 'mental health concerns' [7] and 'mental health problems [8–10].

During this chapter reference will be restricted to persons taken into police custody settings. A detainee generally, but not always, is someone who has been arrested in connection with an offence, taken to a police station and placed before a custody officer. Consideration will be given to provisions for two main groups, first, those people taken to a police custody office as a 'place of safety' using the emergency powers available under s136 Mental Health Act, (MHA) 1983. It is important to recognise those detained, for this reason may not have committed any offences [11]; this power is for the purposes of assessment for their health and wellbeing and to ensure the safety of others. The main focus will be on such detainees.

R. McGrath (✉)
University of Teesside, Middlesbrough, UK
e-mail: Ruth.McGrath@tees.ac.uk

© The Author(s), under exclusive license to Springer Nature
Switzerland AG 2023
T. Scott (ed.), *Mental Health: Intervention Skills for the Emergency Services*,
https://doi.org/10.1007/978-3-031-20347-3_4

The second group encompasses those detainees arrested on suspicion of committing an offence (referred to as 'suspects'), who subsequently, during detention, exhibit evidence they may be experiencing mental ill-health. Whilst two quite separate groups of detainees, many of the processes relating to their care whilst detained are similar. Thus, it is not always possible to distinguish between the two groups. Discussion within the chapter is focused on the adult detainee, i.e. over 18 years, whilst acknowledging that those under the age of 18 years are regarded as vulnerable persons and afforded additional care and observation during detention and interviewing.

Concepts discussed as the chapter progresses include the meaning of police custody and arguments against the use of a police station as a 'place of safety' for people with mental ill-health. Police custody has risks for detainees, and some consideration is given to the healthcare needs of those in custody, together with safeguards in place for vulnerable persons in the investigative process. In the later stages, recent changes to policing detainees with mental ill-health and diversion schemes to minimise risks to individuals will be discussed.

Throughout the chapter there will be reference to relevant legislation and guidance determining the treatment of those detained by police for either of these reasons. In particular reference will be made to:

- *Mental Health Act* [3] (MHA) and its Code of Practice
- *The Mental Health Act* [12] *(Places of Safety) Regulations 2017*
- Police and Criminal Evidence Act [5] (PACE) and Code C
- Policing and Crime Act [13] (PCA)
- Human Rights Act [14] (HRA)

It is suggested that following the large-scale deinstitutionalisation of mental health services in the 1980s, there was a notable increase in the number of contacts between police officers and those with mental health disorders [2]. This is compounded by the fact that such a contact sometimes requires extended time commitments to facilitate an effective response and the recognition that many are repeated contacts [15]. It is acknowledged there are a multitude of triggers underpinning mental ill-health, including substance abuse [16]. In the context of this chapter, this is an important point, as operational police officers recognise increasing links between substance abuse and mental ill-health amongst those they encounter daily. A 2012 localised study of risk assessments completed by Custody Sergeants in Northumbria indicated almost 22% of detainees had a mental health problem [9].

The protection of life is a consideration underpinning every decision taken by a police officer, yet dealing with the needs of vulnerable persons, particularly those with mental health disorders, has only relatively recently become a significant part of the police training curriculum [1]. The absence of training is identified as a potential cause of under-identification of detainees with mental health problems in the custody setting [17]. This training need was highlighted in the multiagency study

At Risk, Yet Dismissed [10] which documents responses from people with mental health problems some of whom experienced lack of understanding in respect of their condition which were perceived as negative encounters with police officers. Further, a joint inspection of policing and mental health recognised that although a range of initiatives were being introduced across police forces to develop the skills of police officers, raising awareness of mental ill-health and appropriate support needs of those they encountered, training was still considered inadequate [11].

The 2014 Mental Health Crisis Care Concordat (CCC) [18] is a national agreement between services and agencies involved in supporting people in crisis. The CCC committed to reviewing existing police training and responses to people with mental ill-health to ensure understanding and updated guidance in the policing environment [18, 19]. A National Strategy published in 2017 recommended regular reviews of mental health training programmes [20] which forms part of the Her Majesty's Inspectorate of Constabulary and Fire and Rescue Service (HMICFRS) inspection process. The inspection process checks every step taken to minimise detainee risk. All actions are closely scrutinised to ensure compliance with guidance and legislation, including PACE 1984, HRA 1998 and in this case, MHA 1983.

2   Police Custody

The care and welfare of those detained at a police station is a specific responsibility of the custody officer, usually a police officer of at least the rank of sergeant [5], incorporating the period of detention, to the stage of charging and release, or other means of disposal. In contrast, the Custody Inspector (sometimes referred to as the PACE Inspector) has responsibility for supervision and support of custody staff and oversight of processes and procedures within the custody environment, which includes ensuring that risks, vulnerabilities and welfare of detainees are managed [21]. This is particularly significant today in respect of s136 Mental Health Act (1983) detentions.

Most people detained on suspicion of having committed an offence are taken to a police station with a custody facility. Inside a custody area, the reason for the arrest is outlined to the custody officer by the arresting or escorting officer. The custody officer will then decide whether or not detention is necessary for further investigation of the offence [5]. Following the decision to authorise detention of suspects, an initial risk assessment is undertaken to assess their fitness for detention. At this point an individual is given an opportunity to disclose any health issues, including those relating to mental health, any medication prescribed and any indicators such as self-harm which may warrant additional support or care whilst in custody. In the event of a disclosure, or subsequent behavioural or health changes being noted, a healthcare professional assessment may determine whether the individual is fit to be detained. During their detention period, their ongoing health is monitored for any change which may require further support or treatment. By contrast, on the arrival of the s136 detainee, the custody officer considers authorising detention for the purpose of medical assessment and will commence the process of arranging the assessment.

3   Police Custody as a 'Place of Safety'

The Mental Health Act (MHA) 1983 (s136 (1)(a) provides the power for a police officer to detain someone if they appear to be suffering from a mental disorder and is in immediate need of care or control. Often referred to as experiencing mental health 'crisis', that person may be removed to a 'place of safety' to enable assessment of immediate mental health needs. Section 135 (6) (MHA 1983) defines the term 'place of safety', explaining which premises might be considered a 'place of safety' which includes hospitals and care homes for those with mental disorders. Perhaps more surprising is the inclusion of police stations, which are not generally designed for use as a 'place of safety', and therefore unable to effectively meet the needs of those individuals suffering from a mental disorder [2].

In 2005/2006 there were 11,517 people held in police detention in England and Wales for the purposes of 'a place of safety' under s136—almost twice the number of those detained in a hospital environment (5900) [22]. When compared with years 2013/2014 to 2015/2016, it can be clearly seen that whilst the scale of those detained under s136 is growing, fewer people were taken to police cells as a 'place of safety', the majority taken to health-based places of safety (Table 1).

The recording of data relating to s136 MHA 1983 detentions was adjusted to ensure transparency and accuracy and was formally collected by the Home Office from 2016/2017 (Table 2); this change of recording may explain the reduction in figures in the year 2016/2017.

Whilst s136 detentions are, in the main, increasing, year on year, the number of detainees taken to police stations as a 'place of safety' is reducing. An exception to this is in the statistics for 2019/2020 which indicates a very slight increase in detainees taken to a police station as a place of safety, although an unchanged percentage. This is not currently a cause for alarm but will be monitored.

The Mental Health Act 1983 (Places of Safety) Regulations 2017 explains when an adult may be kept at a police station as 'place of safety' for the purposes of s135 and s136 of the Mental Health Act 1983. This will only occur when it is believed their behaviour presents an immediate risk of serious injury or death to themselves

Table 1 Number of Section 136 detentions in England and Wales 2013 to 2016 [23]

	Total s136 to police cells	Total taken by police to health-based places of safety	Total
2013/2014	6667	19,470	26,137
2014/2015	4537	19,065	23,602
2015/2016	2100	26,171	28,271

or others; there is no alternative place of safety in the area; and they will have access

Table 2 Section 136 Mental Health Act 1983 detentions [24–27]

	Section 136 detentions taken to police station	Taken to health-based places of safety (including A&E)	Taken to other place of safety, (including private home/not known)	Total Section 136 detentions by police
2016/2017	1029 (4%)	22,379	2920	26,328
2017/2018	471 (2%)	26,657	2534	29,662
2018/2019	136 (0.5%)	29,080	4022	33,238
2019/2020	159 (0.5%)	29,518	4566	34,243

to a healthcare professional whilst detained at the police station. This detention was, until 2017, for a period of up to 72 hours, considerably longer than for a criminal offence without charge. However, the Policing and Crime Act [13] amended s138 of the *MHA 1983*, reducing the maximum period for detention in a place of safety to 24-h, which could possibly be extended by a further 12 hours in specific circumstances.

Prior to this change, the case of MS v UK [28] highlighted a situation in which MS was detained during a period of crisis and, owing to the absence of an appropriate healthcare setting, was detained in a police station for a period of time exceeding 72-h before health services located a medium secure bed. The European Court of Human Rights concluded that although the initial detention was valid and lawful and the only available option in the circumstances, Article 3 of the *European Convention on Human Rights* had been violated by police (Prohibition of Torture) [29], in particular in relation to the forced medical treatment received during the detention, despite there being no intention by police to degrade MS. This case emphasised the unsuitability of police stations as a place of safety.

Reasons for detention under s136 are documented as including attempting suicide, self-harm, paranoia or showing signs of extreme confusion [11], none of which, it is suggested, are situations which can be effectively dealt with in a police custody environment. Many examples exist of people requiring professional help, instead being placed in a police cell, on 'suicide watch' (under close proximity observation) rather than being in the care of trained health professionals [30] however, Home Office figures shown above indicate clearly this practice is less likely to occur as the number of s136 detentions in police cells reduce.

Police officers have long expressed frustration when attempting to resolve situations involving people with mental ill-health who are unable to get the support they need in the community. They may be faced with detaining someone who appears to be in immediate need of care rather than detention and have to take them to a police station as a 'place of safety' because alternative options are unavailable at that time, as in the case of MS v UK. Police Officers themselves do not believe that police custody is an appropriate place for those with mental ill-health [11]. Later this chapter highlights changes which have been implemented in recent years to overcome this situation, influenced by the CCC, and again highlighted by the report 'Picking up the Pieces' [31].

4   Risk Factors in Police Custody

When police officers engage in a s136 detention, they are responsible for arranging transportation to a 'place of safety'. Where transportation is via ambulance, there should also be a police escort to ensure safe handover (16.41 MHA 1983 Code of Practice).

It is important to note that the PCA [13] introduced a new s136 (1c) to the *MHA 1983*, which requires a police officer to consult a healthcare professional before removing a person to a place of safety. This is referred to later when discussing Street Triage. An officer of at least the rank of inspector will give authority, once all other options have been carefully explored for the detainee to be taken to the police station [32]. Evidence of this effect was recently demonstrated by a police officer who commented on how the custody officer now asks additional questions about all detainees prior to their arrival at the custody office to establish whether there is need to divert to a facility other than a police station. Granting authority to attend the police office with a s136 detainee is now a rarer event.

Similarly, authorising the detention of a s136 detainee in the custody setting is carefully considered and undertaken with due regard to all the circumstances, ensuring the removal of liberty is appropriate, and again requires consultation with a healthcare professional. Ongoing care of that person and any detainee suspected of a crime is a responsibility carefully monitored and documented. Detainees often have health problems which need the attention of a healthcare professional during their detention period. The detainee displaying mental ill-health may also have other medical issues, perhaps requiring the administration of medicine or even emergency department (ED) attention [9].

It is fair to say that the greatest fear of the custody officer concerns a detainee dying whilst in their care, a situation which unfortunately sometimes occurs. As some forms of mental health illness are drug-related and the number of drug-dependent detainees grows, there are realistic concerns for the safety of those individuals, who may also be fragile mentally or physically. One factor to consider is that whilst healthcare professionals can administer specific prescribed drugs, this is not possible in every case, owing to the risk of producing an overdose from a drugs cocktail.

A detailed longitudinal study (1998–2009) was undertaken by the then Independent Police Complaints Commission (IPCC), analysing data relating to the incidence of deaths in (or following) police custody [33]. One area examined indicated deaths related to the mental health and suicide of detainees. Of 95 deaths during those 11 years, 17 people had been detained by police under s136 Mental Health

Act, 1983, 9 being taken to police custody as a 'place of safety', rather than a hospital or other healthcare facility. Two subjects were detained under other sections of the Mental Health Act, 1983, and 39 people were identified as having possible mental health needs at the time of, or following, their arrest. Eleven had been identified as being at risk of suicide or self-harm, and another 26 were not identified as being at risk but went on to commit suicide [33].

The IPCC, now the Independent Office for Police Conduct (IOPC), continues to collate statistics relating to deaths of those detained in police custody. In the period 2020/2021, 19 people died in (or following) police custody in England and Wales. Of those, 12 had mental health concerns, 2 were specifically detained under the Mental Health Act 1983 and 1 death occurring during transportation to hospital; the second had arrived at hospital and was still under police guard when he backed himself out of a window [34]. It is noted that the statistical categories on causes of death do not reveal multiple factors, e.g. the person with known mental ill-health, who has perhaps consumed both drugs and alcohol. This means that figures can sometimes be less reliable than they appear at first sight.

5   Healthcare Needs

Section 136 of The Mental Health Act 1983 provides for individuals to be removed to a place of safety by the police for the purpose of assessment. This is explained by the Code of Practice [35], which specifies from the outset a police station should only be used as a 'place of safety' in exceptional circumstances (Code of Practice 16.38). It is recognised that police cells are inappropriate places to detain people with mental health problems if there are other appropriate alternatives. The new s136A(1) *MHA 1983* specifies that a police station may only be used as a 'place of safety' for those aged 18 and over. Policing guidance reinforces this [24, 36]. Regarding s136 detainees, the greater concern is for their welfare and/or self-harm risk.

Occasionally, it may be necessary for adults to be detained in a police station, as defined in the *MHA (Places of Safety) Regulations (2017)*, but these should be exceptional circumstances. Primarily this would include occasions when it is necessary to regard a police station as a 'place of safety', where there is a considered and imminent risk of serious injury or death to that person, or another, and that there is no alternative place of safety which can reasonably be expected to detain the adult, perhaps because there is not a more suitable alternative immediately available, as was the situation in MS v the UK. In this event it is required that a medical examination be undertaken as soon as possible following arrival at the police station (*MHA 1983 Code of Practice 16.44*). Now, each police area has agreements with the local health authority establishing maximum periods of time an individual will wait before being assessed (or transferred to a more suitable place of safety) by the appropriate health and social care professionals. During this period there should be ongoing healthcare presence available, with checks every half hour by a healthcare professional accordance with Regulation 4 (*MHA (Places of Safety) Regulations, 2017*).

It must be remembered that the s136 detainee is not necessarily suspected of committing a criminal offence. Many detainees suspected of criminal offences may be subsequently found to have mental health issues once accepted into custody. Staff are directly responsible for observing and supervising detainees. To do so they need to be adequately briefed regarding any risks identified and of the level of supervision required for each detainee. Whilst the initial examination is in accordance with the requirements of *PACE Code C* (paras 9.5, 9.5a, 9.5b, note 9c) and MHA 1983, it is important that the outcomes of any such examinations are recorded, necessary documentation completed and relevant staff apprised of the outcomes, particularly where detention continues. Should a suspect be transferred temporarily for hospital attention, this documentation should be taken with them to ensure everyone involved in their custody or care is fully informed.

Most police forces have access to an on-call adult healthcare professional 24-h a day. However, such staff may not all have specific mental health training. Where there are concerns a suspect may be experiencing mental ill-health, the on-call crisis team will be contacted to attend the custody area to assess the individual. In accordance with *PACE Code C*, until proved otherwise, the suspect will be considered to be a vulnerable person and treated accordingly. This recognition of needs is relatively recent, one consideration being that a person with mental ill-health may perceive themselves to be regarded as a criminal—being placed in a cell, on occasions being placed under constant surveillance to ensure they do not harm themselves [2].

As recently as 2013, people taken to police stations as a 'place of safety' underwent the same processes as other detainees in terms of being 'booked in' and undergoing a risk assessment before being placed in a cell and locked in [11]. It is recognised that being in police custody increases emotional uncertainty, particularly for a first-time detainee. The environment is hostile, with detainees often subjected to continuous shouting and banging from other detainees [37], whilst the limited space reinforces the sense of captivity, and the procedures a detainee undergoes, e.g. taking fingerprints, removal of personal belongings, etc., emphasise the power balance in favour of the police [38] whilst reinforcing the punitive effect of custody [39]. This process can be difficult for anyone, but for a s136 detainee, it can emphasise the feeling of being treated as a criminal, rather than as a person needing help, which may be detrimental to their welfare [19].

Any interaction with a detainee must be recorded by the relevant member of staff, to include any visits and observations, the detainee's behaviour or condition and any changes to that as time progresses.

There are four levels of observation outlined by the College of Policing [40]:

- *Level 1*: General Observation—the minimum accepted level of observation for any detainee post-risk assessment, which includes checks at least hourly during the detention period.
- *Level 2*: Intermittent Observation—the minimum accepted level for detainees under the influence of alcohol or drugs, which includes checks at least every 30 mins.

- *Level 3*: Constant Observation—undertaken where a risk assessment indicates a heightened level of risk to the detainee. This includes self-harm, suicide risk or other significant mental or physical vulnerability. Here constant observation may be via CCTV cell monitoring, but physical checks again will be at least every 30 mins, possible ligatures will be removed and the individual will be reviewed by a healthcare practitioner.
- *Level 4*: Close Proximity—this applies to those detainees at the highest risk of self-harm and includes physical supervision in close proximity to enable immediate physical intervention where necessary. (This observation level is sometimes referred to as 'suicide watch').

Observations are undertaken in accordance with PACE Code C Annex H that outlines criteria to be considered during the observation visit which would give further cause for concern and prompt examination by a healthcare professional or the calling of an ambulance. Detainees displaying mental ill-health are more likely to be observed at Level 3 or perhaps Level 4 if other indications of risk are present. The custody officer will be involved in the ongoing risk assessment of an individual and can adjust the observation level in accordance with an increase or decrease in risk. However, from the perspective of a custody officer, it is preferable to have a police officer sitting in a crisis centre for 4 h with a detainee than to undertake close proximity observation in a custody suite. Particularly concerning the s136 detainee, this will avert deprivation of their liberty, whilst they are in the least harmful environment, minimising risk to them.

Where a detainee is already prescribed medication, this information will be recorded at the point of the initial risk assessment incorporated into documentation procedures when first accepted into custody. Any medication accompanying the detainee will be recorded and put in a safe place. Prior to the medication being administered, the custody officer will consult the healthcare professional. The nature of the medication will determine its administration, in accordance with the Misuse of Drugs Regulations (MDR), 2001 [41], but also with reference to other indicators, including behaviour and physical appearance. This acknowledges the adjustments considered in view of the increasing number of detainees with mental ill-health affected by drug abuse, which in some cases will raise concerns as to the safety of administering already prescribed medication.

6   Vulnerability and the Investigation

Since being updated in 2019, *PACE 1984 Code C* now incorporates a wider definition of vulnerability [42] which is important in the situation of the detainee suspected of an offence and the ongoing formal investigative processes that would necessarily be undertaken post arrest, commencing with the interview. The definition of vulnerability in respect of detainees has been subject of debate. A 2016 study of custody officers asked them to define the term 'vulnerability'. Participants tended to construct their own definition, rather than using that contained in Code C of

PACE 1984. Recommendations included use of the precise list of specific conditions contained in MHA 1983 Code of Practice by police officers [43]. It is argued that such an approach would not necessarily recognise the many different forms of vulnerability and also that at different points in their lives, many people could be regarded as vulnerable, for a range of reasons [44]. Therefore, a tight definition may be less helpful in responding to individual needs.

Since the 2016 research Code C has been updated (2019). Although it does refer to other forms of vulnerability, it states 'A person may be vulnerable as a result of having a mental health condition or mental disorder' (Note 1G). It further explains that where an officer has reason to suspect a person may be vulnerable as a result of a mental health condition or mental disorder, they should be regarded as vulnerable until there is clear evidence to dispel that suspicion. In order to establish the vulnerability of a person, there should be reasonable enquiries to acquire information, record any factors to support this belief and ensure that anyone coming into contact with the individual is made aware of that record (1.4; Annex E).

Guidance for managing the detention of vulnerable persons has also been updated [40]. It provides for those circumstances where a vulnerable person may have difficulty in understanding fully the implications of the processes; they may be subject to (1.13 (d) (i) (ii)), or become confused, or provide unreliable or incriminating information (iii). Establishing this may emerge from information disclosed by the individual during the initial risk assessment, or subsequently whilst in custody (in 2009), the reliance on self-reporting meant that actual statistics indicating the number of detainees with mental health disorders was unreliable [8]; information may be supplied by family members or associates; there may be existing knowledge of the individual via previous encounters; it may emerge following examination with a healthcare professional or Approved Mental Health Professional (AMHP). However, it is important to remember that whilst mental health carers or other agencies working in the community may be able to supply information, the individual may not be known to those services [36].

In the late 1980s, mental health encounters were often the source of frustration for police officers recognising the need to support individuals, but with neither the skills nor capacity to offer that support. As an example, a police officer recalled an offence of arson, in which both social services and a doctor having spoken with the detainee declared him to have a 'personality defect'. The detainee's explanation and other supporting evidence suggested a more serious mental health disorder, yet the outcome was that the defendant was charged with the offence, convicted at court and released into the community again, without further support ([45]: 169). By 2009 little had altered, police having no standard mental health assessment and little training around mental health awareness [8]. This illustrates some of the difficulties experienced by the police in this time period and for the next two decades.

7   Appropriate Adult

Code C of *PACE 1984* (1.7) establishes and defines the role of the Appropriate Adult in relation to the safeguarding of rights, entitlements and welfare of vulnerable persons suspected of crime. This includes supporting and advising the vulnerable person when asked to participate in procedures such as interviews, observing whether the police are acting properly and fairly and helping the individual to understand their rights, and to communicate with the police if they wish to do so (2019). There is a requirement for a custody officer to inform the Appropriate Adult as soon as reasonably practicable of the grounds for detention and the location of the detainee and secure the attendance of an Appropriate Adult to see the detainee (Annex E, 2019). Whilst the presence of the Appropriate Adult during an interview safeguards their rights, it is noted that the role supports the progression of the judicial processes, i.e. ensuring an interview takes place, and that any evidence arising from that will be admissible in court. The emphasis is on fairness, rather than the mental health needs of those involved [2].

The Appropriate Adult may know the detainee—they may be a relative, guardian or other person responsible for their care or custody, or they may be another, independent, person. Today police forces have access to trained Appropriate Adults where it is not possible to use someone known to the detainee. Bradley identified that the provision of access to Appropriate Adults was inconsistent across police forces, suggesting that detainees with mental ill-health might not all have opportunity to receive the same level of support. It recommended a review of the Appropriate Adult role and the provision of additional training to ensure the police provide effective support for detainees ([8]: 43).

By 2014 it was established that progress in respect of access to Appropriate Adults was 'slow'. At times Appropriate Adults were not available to support detainees, and there was evidence that Appropriate Adults were not always requested by custody staff. It was also recognised that training for Appropriate Adults was available, but not subscribed to by all providers across England and Wales [19, 37].

A decade later the follow-up report *In Ten Years' Time* recognised the developments enshrined in Code C, yet noted ongoing issues with the recognition of vulnerability, again questioning the extent of access to an Appropriate Adult by some detainees [46]. The Mental Health charity 'Mind' now operates a rotation service for Appropriate Adults, in agreement with many local police forces. They manage a pool of volunteers with police station training and when contacted by custody office will make arrangements for someone to attend when required, to support the necessary police procedures. A further safeguard, in accordance with PACE 1984, is the role of Independent Custody Visitors (ICV), local volunteers who visit custody officers to check that detainees are receiving rights and entitlements and that their well-being and dignity is being upheld whilst in custody. They also check if there is timely provision of Appropriate Adults, to avoid extension of detention time as a result of having to wait for their attendance [47]. This can be seen as a safeguard both for the detainee and for the custody officer.

8   The Changing Face of Policing People with Mental Ill-Health

Table 3 below offers a brief timeline covering the period 2012 to 2018 of mental health legislation and policy changes impacting on procedures relating to detainees with mental ill-health. This table does not include every inquiry or review or change in legislation but shows the development of change during the course of a decade.

As alluded to in the early stages of this chapter, policing approaches to the care of detainees with mental ill-health have changed in recent years. One of the key factors in the change process was the signing of the CCC in 2014, a recognition by many signatory partners that those experiencing mental ill-health should be given greater support in times of crisis [18]. For the first time, this showed a common willingness and commitment to make long-term changes to provision for those in need of specialised support, at every stage of their encounter with services.

The *Policing Vision 2025* recognised that the police service needed to increase its understanding of the needs of vulnerable persons, including those with mental ill-health, and to develop its practices by engaging in partnerships with other services to provide the care and support needed [50]. Evidence of application of these recommendations can be seen in a range of training initiatives for police officers and staff. Examples include one partnership between the Tees, Esk and Wear Valleys NHS Foundation Trust (TEWV) and Cleveland Police, which incorporates awareness training for police officers, led by trained Mental Health Nurses. This is considered to be good practice and offers an enhanced training approach [51]. The subsequent CCC Evaluation Report identified other specific areas of training being undertaken for police officers, including training on autism, suicide awareness and suicide prevention training, training on self-harm for ED staff and raising awareness of the links between substance misuse and self-harming behaviour as well as working with dual diagnosis more generally [19]. More recently an initiative in Nottinghamshire Police facilitates probationary officers to work for a day in a mental health setting to increase their awareness and understanding of mental ill-health, whilst North Yorkshire Police work in collaboration to provide multiagency training for all staff [7].

The National Strategy for Police Custody [20] encompassed the changing approach of the police service to the topic of mental health. This report again acknowledged that whilst police custody could offer access to mental health support, it was not necessarily the most appropriate response when dealing with incidents relating to mental ill-health, recommending that such detention is no longer carried out in police custody facilities. The success of this report can be seen in the statistics shown earlier in this chapter, which indicates a major shift away from the use of the police station as a 'place of safety' to the use of other healthcare settings more appropriate to the needs of individuals [24–27].

Table 3 Timeline of mental health legislation and policy changes 2012 to 2018

2012	MS v UK the important ruling by the European Court of Human Rights that although MS had been detained appropriately and lawfully, his detention at a police station which exceeded 7-h breached Article 3 of the Convention
2012	Street Triage projects commence
2013	*Independent Commission on Mental Health and Policing Report* [48] published following the review of the Metropolitan Police Service (MPS) at the request of the Metropolitan Police Commissioner. Made a series of recommendations specific to the MPS but which influenced thinking at a national level
2014	The signing of the Mental Health Crisis Care Concordat (CCC) by 22 services and agencies involved in the care and support of people in crisis
2015	House of Commons Home Affairs Committee Report HC 202 *Policing and Mental Health House of Commons (2015)* Recommended a series of changes including: • The commissioning of additional health-based places of safety by July 2015 • Using police cells as a place of safety only in extreme situations—and not for children • Expansion of Street Triage schemes and a full evaluation • Liaison and diversion schemes • Improved training for police officers and staff • Amendment to *MHA 1983* to reduce detention time from 72 hours to 24 hours maximum
2017	*Report of the Independent Review of Deaths and Serious Incidents in Police Custody* [49] focuses on all deaths in custody but recommendations in relation to mental health: • National, comprehensive, quality assured mental health training for all officers in front-line or custody roles • Reinforces that police stations are not appropriate places of safety for those suffering from an acute mental health crisis • Recommends funding of Liaison and Diversion Schemes and Street Triage • Consistent guidance for police to ensure an improved policing approach to those in mental health need • Use of police vehicles for transporting those detained under s136 should cease • Use of police stations as places of safety should be phased out
2017	Policing and Crime Act [13]—amended the *Mental Health Act 1983* re: • Extension of powers under s135 and s136 (searching for and removal of persons) • Consultation of relevant health professional prior to removal to and detention at place of safety • Restrictions on places used as a place of safety • Prohibits children being taken to a police station as a place of safety • Reduces maximum periods of detention under s136 to 24 hours and establishes reasons for extending detention for a further maximum of 12 hours • Establishes protective searches of detainees
2018	HMICFRS (2018) Report *Policing and Mental Health: Picking up the Pieces*—Assessment of how effective forces are at protecting and helping those with mental health problems. Main recommendations: • Development of a new national definition of mental ill-health for policing • Evaluation of mental health demand, triage services, training programmes

9   Diversion from Police Custody

The CCC evaluation incorporated research undertaken during 2015 with people who had been subject to crisis care. Some identified more positive interactions with the police than in previous encounters, one person making positive references to being placed in a 'witness room' outside the custody suite, rather than in a cell whilst detained [19]. Unfortunately, few police stations are able to provide specialist facilities, thus reinforcing the need for alternative healthcare provision, one indicating they use a separate wing of the custody block for these purposes to minimise contact with other detainees and reduce noise levels a little.

Reference has already been made to the amendments applied to the *MHA* 1983 following the introduction of the *PCA 2017*, which extended powers under s135 and s136. One amendment requires police to consult, where possible, with a healthcare professional before applying s136. Street Triage schemes offer one way in which this consultation or assessment may be achieved and is intended to reduce the need to invoke s136 *MHA 1983*, diverting those with mental health issues from police custody and also hospitals, to provide appropriate care for their needs

An initial small-scale pilot study of Street Triage, commencing in 2012, was extended in 2015 to additional forces on the recommendation of the report *Policing and Mental Health* [52], and by 2018, 42 of the 43 police forces were operating a Street Triage system in partnership with other agencies. Street Triage operates differently from force to force, but examples include the use of police vehicles containing mental health professionals in the crew, who respond directly to incidents, locating mental healthcare professionals in control rooms to advise operational officers and the availability of helplines to speak with specialist mental health nurses [31]. One NHS Foundation trust works in partnership with two police forces, providing a team of mental health nurses to support local Street Triage processes by providing a rapid assessment to assist the decision-making process and determine the most appropriate response [51]. This process reduces the number of people being held in custody under *MHA 1983* [53].

Anecdotally, a police officer reported their experiences of Street Triage, noting that in their police force, between 08.00 and 20.00, a police officer works with a registered mental health nurse, and then further support is available out of hours via their control room. A study in the Northumbria Police area indicated links between the use of Street Triage and a reduction in s136 detentions when using Street Triage processes [54]. Another force reported a 57% reduction in the use of s136 detentions between 2011/2012 and 2016/2017 as a direct use of Street Triage [55].

An example of where Street Triage could be very effective can be seen in the case of an agitated individual, with mental health issues, who storms out of the home stating they are going to kill themself and then proceeds to run in and out of traffic risking both their life and that of other road users, a situation similar to that of James Herbert [23]. In this situation police officers at one time might have considered the only powers of arrest available to them are for a Breach of the Peace, in order to ensure the physical wellbeing of the individual. Today a more appropriate response would be to engage with the Street Triage process which would enable a rapid assessment of the individual's needs and ultimately lead to alternative healthcare solutions.

Earlier in this chapter, reference was made to IPCC data showing the numbers of people taken to police cells in 2013/2014 as s136 detainees were as high as 6667. It is pleasing to see the change in policing approaches. Today s136 detainees are taken to police stations as a last resort. In 2013 the custody officer alone took the decision as to whether or not to accept the detainee into that 'place of safety'. Today a police station is considered a last resort, an individual being housed there only on the authority of a more senior officer, usually the Custody Inspector, who is responsible for PACE detainees. This authority is generally given only when an alternative mental health establishment is unable to house the individual, an example of this being where evidence indicates their violent behaviour is putting others at risk. It is notable that where a detainee is refused admission to hospital, or treatment by ambulance staff, the police retain a duty of care for them. As such they must, where possible, ensure the detainee is examined and assessed [21]. It is important to remember that no detainee regarded as a vulnerable person should be released from custody without first being subject of a prerelease risk assessment. During this risk assessment, the custody officer will check that all relevant support has been made available to them during their detention. This is part of the process of ensuring there will be support from other agencies in place to protect their wellbeing when finally released.

10   Diversion from the Broader Criminal Justice System

The Bradley Report [8] outlined the findings of the independent review in relation to diverting offenders with mental health problems from prison and indeed to establish how early interventions might prevent vulnerable children and adults entering the criminal justice system. The report identified that closer working relationships between the police and health and social services could avoid prosecution of those with mental disorders.

This led to the introduction of liaison and diversion schemes, intended to ensure people with mental ill-health who enter the criminal justice system have access to early assessment to identify their needs at the earliest opportunity. In terms of the policing process this can involve the following:

- A decision taken not to invoke the criminal law, e.g. by not taking any further action against the individual or by discontinuing a prosecution
- Diversion from prosecution by use of a fixed penalty notice, or caution or community resolution [21, 56].

Here decisions about diversion are taken by the police and the CPS and may also involve other agencies; however, the police duty of care does not stop here and often leads to referral to another agency for ongoing support for the individual. Some police forces have a mental health diversion team based in the custody area, comprising mental health nurses and triage staff, who are able to put support in place at an early point in their custody. It is important to recognise the distinction between their role and that of the crisis team who will undertake s136 assessment and make the decision as to whether the individual can safely remain in a custody environment.

11   Conclusion

Approaches to the police detention of those experiencing mental ill-health have changed, particularly during the last decade, but this has occurred only with the benefit of collaborative approaches to change across relevant services. The deinstitutionalisation of mental health services in the 1980s led to an increased demand on the police service, yet there was no corresponding recognition of this in terms of appropriate training or support resources.

This chapter focused on detainees with mental health issues, primarily those detained under s36 *MHA* 1983, and did not discuss police actions in the wider community. However, it is clear that a growing movement of concern for those with mental health needs has impacted on the role of the police officer in the public arena, and within the custody setting, and during the last decade, this has led to a shift in approaches, in particular, in the reduced number of those detained in a police station and the reduction of deaths in custody of detainees in crisis.

The work undertaken to increase the support for vulnerable persons has contributed to the important revisions to the *Mental Health Act 1983* via the Policing and Crime Act [13], to ensure the welfare of those detainees in the custody process. No longer is a police custody area considered to be an appropriate 'place of safety' for anyone under 18. Those over 18 cannot be taken to a police station as a 'place of safety', without consultation with a health professional and then the authorisation of an inspector, and only ever as a last resort. Most important, is the revised period of detention, now only 24 hours rather than the previous 72 hours.

The reduction in numbers of s136 detainees in police stations is evident from Home Office statistics. This in turn reduces the pressure upon the custody staff to ensure the welfare of other detainees, many of whom will also have mental ill-health. It is too early to tell whether this has had a significant impact on deaths in custody of detainees with mental ill-health.

Existing provisions in place for medical attention for detainees did not necessarily respond to mental health needs. Custody staff are now trained to recognise indicators of risk of self-harming or of mental health needs requiring a greater level of care than other detainees. Additionally, access to appropriate medical healthcare practitioners has now been established and is proving effective, and with a focus on early assessment of needs, risks can be greatly reduced and the current four-stage observation levels formally establish where additional care is required in the context of the individual. Amendments to *Code C* of *PACE 1984* have updated this important guidance for custody staff, putting in place stronger safeguarding measures to ensure fairness and consideration of needs throughout the process, yet recognising when police custody is no longer an appropriate measure. This becomes ever more important with increases in detainees with mental ill-health related to drug misuse.

During the last decade, the provisions associated with the Appropriate Adult scheme have been strengthened to ensure that vulnerable detainees have the protections they need, particularly in relation to the interviewing process, although, as noted, this is a safeguard aimed at ensuring process more than an individual's welfare [2]. The growing use of diversion and liaison schemes indicate recognition that policing is not only about punishment, showing much more consideration to individual circumstances and needs, selecting the most appropriate outcome, with the emphasis on support. Changes outlined in this chapter are refreshing to see, but long overdue, and the custody process should not be considered to be without its issues. The difference between s136 detentions in 2006 (11,500) and in 2020 (159) shows pleasing progress and indicates that appropriate mental healthcare is more readily available to those most in need of it. It is a positive change to note that even in situations where a detainee in crisis is violent, and police station cells are used as a last resort, such detention will not, in the main, exceed 24 hours.

Learning Points
- Outline changes in legislation and policing policy to support detainees displaying mental ill-health symptoms and identify who is responsible for the care and welfare of a detainee in a police custody setting.
- Explain the circumstances for a Section 136 detainee to be held in a police custody setting and how this differs from a person detained on suspicion of a criminal offence.
- Consider what measures must be put in place when a person who displays mental health issues is detained in police custody.

References

1. College of Policing. Authorised Professional Practice. Operations: core planning principles. 2018. https://www.college.police.uk/app/operations/operationalplanning/core-planning-principles. Accessed 15 Jan 2023.
2. Cummins I. A place of safety? Self-harming behaviour in police custody. J Adult Protect. 2008;10(1):36–47.
3. Mental Health Act. 1983. Mental Health Act 1983 (legislation.gov.uk). Accessed 20 Dec 2020.
4. Home Office. Police and Criminal Evidence Act 1984. (PACE): Code G (2012). 2012. https://assets.publishing.service.gov.uk/government/uploads/system/uploads/attachment_data/file/903814/pace-code-g-2012.pdf. Accessed 31 Jan 2022.
5. Police and Criminal Evidence Act. Police and Criminal Evidence Act 1984 (legislation.gov.uk). 1984. Accessed 20 Dec 2020.
6. Home Office. Police and Criminal Evidence Act 1984 (PACE): Code C, revised, code of practice for the detention, treatment and questioning of persons by Police Officers. London: TSO; 2019.

7. Independent Office for Police Conduct. Learning the Lessons: Mental Health 34. 2019. https://www.policeconduct.gov.uk/sites/default/files/Documents/Learningthelessons/34/ LearningtheLessons_Issue34_February_2019.pdf. Accessed 6 Jan 2021.
8. Bradley LK. The Bradley report: Lord Bradley's review of people with mental health problems or learning disabilities in the criminal justice system. London: Department of Health; 2009.
9. Sirdifield C, Brooker C. Detainees in police custody: results of a health needs assessment in Northumbria, England. Int J Prison Health. 2012;8(2):60–7.
10. Victim Support and Mind. At Risk, Yet Dismissed: The criminal victimisation of people with mental health problems. 2013. https://www.mind.org.uk/media-a/4121/at-risk-yet-dismissed-report.pdf. Accessed 3 Dec 2021.
11. Justice Inspectorates. A criminal use of police cells? The use of police custody as a place of safety for people with mental health needs. 2013. https://www.justiceinspectorates.gov.uk/hmicfrs/media/a-criminal-use-of-police-cells-20130620.pdf. Accessed 3 Mar 2021.
12. Mental Health Act. (Places of Safety) Regulations 2017. Available at: The Mental Health Act 1983 (Places of Safety) Regulations 2017 (legislation.gov.uk). 1983. Accessed 20 Dec 2020.
13. Policing and Crime Act. 2017. Policing and Crime Act 2017 (legislation.gov.uk). Accessed 23 Dec 2020.
14. Human Rights Act. 1998. Human Rights Act 1998 (legislation.gov.uk). Accessed: 23 Dec 2020.
15. Kane E, Evans E. Mental health and policing interventions: implementation and impact. Ment Health Rev J. 2018;23(2):86–93. https://doi.org/10.1108/MHRJ-10-2017-0046.
16. National Institute on Drug Abuse. 'Part 1: The Connection Between Substance Use Disorders and Mental Illness'. 2020. https://www.drugabuse.gov/publications/research-reports/common-comorbidities-substance-use-disorders/part-1-connection-between-substance-use-disorders-mental-illness. Accessed 28 Jan 2021.
17. Cummins I. Mental health and custody: a follow on study. J Adult Protect. 2012;14(2):73–81. https://doi.org/10.1108/14668201211217521.
18. HM Government. Mental Health Crisis Care Concordat: Improving Outcomes for People Experiencing Mental Health Crisis. 2014. https://assets.publishing.service.gov.uk/government/uploads/system/uploads/attachment_data/file/281242/36353_Mental_Health_Crisis_accessible.pdf. Accessed 5 Jan 2021.
19. Gibson S, Hamilton S, James K. Evaluation of the crisis care Concordat: Final Report. 2016. https://s16878.pcdn.co/wp-content/uploads/2016/03/CCC-Evaluation_Report.pdf. Accessed 30 Dec 2020.
20. National Police Chiefs' Council. National Strategy for Police Custody. 2017. https://www.npcc.police.uk/documents/NPCC%20Custody%20Strategy.pdf. Accessed 24 Dec 2020.
21. College of Policing. Authorised Professional Practice. Detainee care: diversion and referral. 2020. https://www.college.police.uk/app/detention-andcustody/detainee-care/detainee-care#diversion-and-referral-58. Accessed 15 Jan 2023.
22. Docking M, Grace K, Bucke T. Police custody as a "Place of Safety": Examining the Use of Section 136 of the Mental Health Act 1983. 2008. https://webarchive.nationalarchives.gov.uk/20100908154141/http://www.ipcc.gov.uk/section_136.pdf. Accessed 3 Jan 2021.
23. Independent Police Complaints Commission (IPCC). Six Missed Chances. 2017. https://www.policeconduct.gov.uk/sites/default/files/Documents/research-learning/James_Herbert_Six_missed_chances.pdf. Accessed 5 Jan 2021.
24. Home Office. Police Powers and Procedures, England and Wales, year ending 31 March 2017. 2017. https://assets.publishing.service.gov.uk/government/uploads/system/uploads/attachment_data/file/658099/police-powers-procedures-mar17-hosb2017.pdf. Accessed 20 Dec 2020.
25. Home Office. Police Powers and Procedures, England and Wales, year ending 31 March 2018. 2018. https://assets.publishing.service.gov.uk/government/uploads/system/uploads/attachment_data/file/751215/police-powers-procedures-mar18-hosb2418.pdf. Accessed 20 Dec 2020.

26. Home Office. Police powers and procedures, England and Wales, year ending 31 March 2019. 2019. https://www.gov.uk/government/statistics/police-powers-and-procedures-england-and-wales-year-ending-31-march-2019. Accessed 20 Dec 2020.

27. Home Office. Police Powers and Procedures, England and Wales, year ending 31 March 2020. Available at: Police powers and procedures, England and Wales, year ending 31 March 2020 second edition - GOV.UK (www.gov.uk). 2020. Accessed 20 Mar 2021.

28. MS v UK [2012] ECHR 804; 2012. MHLO 46.

29. Council of Europe. European Convention on Human Rights. Updated Version (2013). 1950. https://www.echr.coe.int/documents/convention_eng.pdf. Accessed 23 Dec 2020.

30. Sutherland J. Crossing the line: lessons from a life on duty. London: Weidenfeld & Nicholson; 2020.

31. Her Majesty's Inspectorate of Constabulary and Fire & Rescue Services. Policing and mental health: picking up the pieces. Policing and mental health: picking up the pieces (justiceinspectorates.gov.uk). 2018. Accessed 2 Jan 2021.

32. Home Office. Guidance for the Implementation of Changes to Police Powers and Places of Safety Provisions in the Mental Health Act, 1983. 2017. https://assets.publishing.service.gov.uk/government/uploads/system/uploads/attachment_data/file/656025/Guidance_on_Police_Powers.PDF. Accessed 5 Jan 2021.

33. Hannan M, Hearnden I, Grace K, Bucke T. Deaths in or following Police custody: an examination of the cases 1998/99-2008/09. IPCC Research Series Paper 17. 2010. https://webarchive.nationalarchives.gov.uk/20170914190041/http://www.ipcc.gov.uk/sites/default/files/Documents/research_stats/Deaths_In_Custody_Report_0811.pdf. Accessed 5 Jan 2021.

34. Independent Office for Police Conduct. Deaths During or Following Police Contact: Statistics for England and Wales, 2020/21. 2021. https://www.policeconduct.gov.uk/sites/default/files/Documents/statistics/deaths_during_following_police_contact_202021.pdf. Accessed 30 July 2021.

35. Dept of Health. Mental health Act 1983: code of practice. London: TSO. 2015. https://assets.publishing.service.gov.uk/government/uploads/system/uploads/attachment_data/file/435512/MHA_Code_of_Practice.PDF. Accessed 2 Jan 2021.

36. College of Policing. Authorised Professional Practice. Mental health detention: relevant definitions. 2020. https://www.college.police.uk/app/mentalhealth/mental-health-detention. Accessed 15 Jan 2023.

37. Leese M, Russell S. Mental health, vulnerability and risk in police custody. J Adult Protect. 2017;19(5):274–83. https://doi.org/10.1108/JAP-03-2017-0006.

38. Wooff A, Skinns L. The role of emotion, space and place in Police custody in England: towards a geography of Police custody. Punishment Soc. 2018;20(5):562–79. https://doi.org/10.1177/1462474517722176.

39. Skinns L, Wooff A, Sprawson A. Preliminary findings on police custody delivery in the twenty-first century: is it 'good' enough? Polic Soc. 2017;27(4):358–71. https://doi.org/10.1080/10439463.2015.1058377.

40. College of Policing. Authorised Professional Practice. Detention and custody: detainee care. 2020. https://www.college.police.uk/app/detention-andcustody/detainee-care/detainee-care. Accessed 15 Jan 2023.

41. HM Government. The Misuse of Drugs Regulations 2001. UK Statutory Instruments 2001 No. 3998 Regulation 1. 2001. https://www.legislation.gov.uk/uksi/2001/3998/regulation/1/made. Accessed 31 Mar 2022.

42. Dehaghani R. Interrogating vulnerability: reframing the vulnerable suspect in police custody. Soc Leg Stud. 2021;30(2):251–71. https://doi.org/10.1177/0964663920921921.

43. Dehaghani R. Custody officers, code C and constructing vulnerability: implications for policy and practice. Policing. 2016;11(1):74–86. https://doi.org/10.1093/police/paw024.

44. Keay S, Kirby S. Defining vulnerability: from the conceptual to the operational. Policing. 2017;12(4):428–38. https://doi.org/10.1093/police/pax046.

45. Graef R. Talking blues: the police in their own words. London: Collins Harvill; 1989.

46. Revolving Doors Agency, and Centre for Mental Health. In Ten Years Time. 2019. Available at: http://www.revolving-doors.org.uk/file/2389/download?token=8M0Vf1U. Accessed 1 Mar 2021.
47. Independent Office for Police Conduct. Learning the lessons: Custody 35. 2019. https://www.policeconduct.gov.uk/sites/default/files/Documents/Learningthelessons/35/LearningtheLessons_Bulletin35_July_2019_single_column.pdf. Accessed 6 Jan 2021.
48. Adebowale V. Independent Commission on Mental Health and Policing. 2013. https://www.basw.co.uk/resources/independent-commission-mental-health-and-policing-report. Accessed 20 Sept 2020.
49. Angiolini E. Independent Review of Deaths and Serious Incidents in Police Custody. 2017. https://assets.publishing.service.gov.uk/government/uploads/system/uploads/attachment_data/file/655401/Report_of_Angiolini_Review_ISBN_Accessible.pdf. Accessed 20 Sept 2020.
50. National Police Chiefs' Council. Policing Vision 2025. 2016. https://www.npcc.police.uk/documents/Policing%20Vision.pdf. Accessed 20 Dec 2020.
51. Tees, Esk and Wear Valleys NHS Foundation Trust. 'Street Triage and Places of Safety'. 2021. https://www.tewv.nhs.uk/services/street-triage-and-places-of-safety/. Accessed 2 Mar 2021.
52. House of Commons, Home Affairs Committee. Policing and Mental Health. Eleventh Report of Session 2014–15. (202). London: HMSO; 2015.
53. Reveruzzi B, Pilling S. Street Triage report on the evaluation of nine pilot schemes in England. 2016. https://s16878.pcdn.co/wp-content/uploads/2016/09/Street-Triage-Evaluation-Final-Report.pdf. Accessed 6 Jan 2021.
54. Keown P, French J, Gibson G, Newton E, Cull S, Brown P, Parry J, Lyons D, McKinnon I. Too much detention? Street triage and detentions under section 136 mental health Act in the northeast of England: a descriptive study of the effects of a Street Triage intervention. BMJ Open. 2016;6:e011837. https://doi.org/10.1136/bmjopen-2016-011837.
55. Cleveland Police. 'Everyone matters equality and diversity report 2017. 2017. https://www.cleveland.police.uk/SysSiteAssets/media/downloads/force-content/cleveland/cp-em-ed-report-2017.pdf. Accessed 5 Jan 2021.
56. National Police Chiefs' Council (NPCC). National Strategy on Policing and Mental Health. 2020. https://www.npcc.police.uk/Mental%20Health/Nat%20Strat%20Final%20v2%2026%20Feb%202020.pdf. Accessed 3 Jan 2021.

Emergency Physician

Catherine Hayhurst

1 Introduction

1.1 Mental Health Presentations to the Emergency Department

Patients presenting to the emergency department (ED) with a mental health problem is a common occurrence. Overall mental health presentations make up around 3–5% of total attendances [1], although many more patients attend who have concurrent mental illness which may affect their ED presentation. Hospital Episode Statistics (HES) for England showed a nearly threefold increase in mental health presentations from 90,079 in 2009/2010 to 266,449 in 2018–2019 [2]. However, subsequent more reliable data from 2019–2022 show steady numbers at around 4% of ED attendances. There are many possible reasons for the measured increase in attendances to 2019, which may have been due to an increase in coding for mental health or there may have been an actual increase in incidence of mental health attendances, or both. A decrease in stigma may have led people in crisis to seek help or lack of community services or a perceived increase in urgency may have pushed people to come to ED rather than seek help elsewhere.

The majority of people presenting to an ED also have an urgent physical health problem such as overdose or self-harm or first presentation of psychosis and so need concurrent physical and mental health assessment and care. During the COVID-19 pandemic, there have been welcome initiatives to provide alternative 24-hour services for people experiencing a crisis in their mental health, such as mental health telephone triage lines and alternative assessment spaces for patients.

C. Hayhurst (✉)
Consultant in Emergency Medicine, Cambridge University Hospitals NHS Foundation Trust, Cambridge, England, UK
e-mail: c.hayhurst@nhs.net

1.2   Patient Views on the ED

Many patients report that the ED environment is a difficult place to be when they are feeling anxious, low, suicidal or agitated. Departments are often crowded and noisy, and staff are stretched as they try to care for each patient. In addition, patients will have mixed feelings about coming to the ED. Some report feeling ashamed of their self-harm, some that they should not be 'wasting our time' or worse they do not deserve care. They may be annoyed that they had to come for treatment or be anxious about what may happen to them whilst they are in our care. For others who have psychotic symptoms, the whole experience can be confusing, disorientating and frightening. Scenario 1 tells of one individual's experience and fears.

Carrie's Experience
Carrie used to come to the ED frequently having taken a large overdose of diphenhydramine and sometimes paracetamol. She took the overdoses to stop herself doing something worse. It would always take her a while to call for help, and when she did, she was initially ambivalent about accepting help, e.g. allowing blood tests, and she found it very hard to talk to ED staff. She often felt that staff were talking about her behind her back. When she was unable to accept blood tests, mostly staff gave her time and sat with her. At other times, she was restrained to facilitate a cannula and blood tests, which she found very distressing. She was able to tell us at one point what helped her accept treatment—giving her time and allowing her to communicate via text rather than speaking. It was clear that she needed reassurance that we would be patient, that we cared about her and that she was in no way wasting our time. After a couple of months of frequent attendance, life got better for Carrie; she was able to go back to work and she stopped coming to the ED.

2   Scenario 1 Carrie's Experience

We learned several things from Carrie:

- The reasons that people self-harm vary.
- Patients can be sensitive to what they perceive are our attitudes.
- Working with someone to find out what helps them is invaluable.
- Sometimes ED is just there to get someone through a crisis in the same way we get people through diabetic or asthmatic crises.

3   What Constitutes Good Care in the ED

Patient experience is a good place to start when considering how to improve care. Kindness is the best descriptor of the attitude needed, added to which effective communication skills are vital. Safety is key at every stage of the patient's journey through ED, and there are features of systems which can turn adequate mental health care into excellent health care. Often, we accept that care for patients with mental health problems is not as good as it can be, rather than aiming for excellent care and excellent systems to support this. Table 1 provides a summary of factors needed to provide good mental health care in the ED. The aim of this chapter is to consider the patient journey through ED outlining kindness, safety and excellent systems of care.

Table 1 A summary of factors needed to provide good mental health care in the ED

KIND	SAFE	EXCELLENT
All staff trained to understand MH issues	Triage	Referral to Psychiatry from triage if fit for assessment
Empathic, staff that listen	Observation	Parallel assessment of physical and mental health needs. Good joint working.
Individual focussed	Safe environment	Calm environment
Leaders as role models	Rapid Tranquilisation protocol	Timely assessment by ED and MH teams
Ask about Mental Health even when primary problem is physical	Joint governance between MH and ED	Plans and case management for Frequent Attenders
	Protocol for when police bring a patient to ED (section 136 England)	Alternative pathways not needing ED

4   Mental Health Triage

The first stage for a patient presenting to the ED with a mental health problem is a conversation with a triage nurse to find out why the patient has come, do a brief risk assessment and plan the ongoing care required. The primary aim is to keep the patient safe whilst they are in the ED. Triage by necessity is short, and it can be challenging to do everything required whilst listening to the patient and providing reassurance that they will receive help.

The mental health input that nurses get in their general training is limited, so directed training in mental health triage should be a requirement before nurses can work at the front door. Training is often best delivered by the mental health team that work in your ED and should include aspects of communication skills and risk assessment. 'Saying what you see' and using this to express empathy can be helpful such as 'You look quite anxious just now. Is there anything we can do to help reduce this?'

Risk assessment involves asking some difficult questions. 'I need to ask you some questions which we ask everyone who comes here after self-harming. Do you have any ongoing thoughts of hurting yourself? Do you feel suicidal right now? Is there a chance you may consider leaving the ED before you get help today?' The responses help determine what level of observation the person needs whilst they are in the ED.

Various systems of triage are available, but none are particularly well validated for use in the ED. The Australian Mental Health Triage Scale is one such example that stratifies patients into five groups according to risk of further self harm or leaving the department before assessment [3, 4].

Triage is only as good as the actions that follow this. The Australian Mental Health Triage Scale identifies the few patients that need to be assessed and treated as an emergency as they are a risk to themselves or others, whilst some require this more urgently to prevent deterioration in their mental state. Triage also should lead front door staff to consider safeguarding issues, to record a physical description of the patient and to search patients at risk of self-harm so that any dangerous items may be removed and to consider where the patient should be placed in the ED. A judgement should be made on the risks and observation should be started according to risk - for example:

- High risk: needing continual 1:1 observation
- Medium risk: needing observations every 15 min
- Low risk: not requiring observation

5 Referral to Mental Health Teams from Triage

An important feature of excellent emergency mental health care is parallel assessment and treatment by ED and mental health clinicians. This is best initiated by a referral from triage to the mental health team working in the ED for any person who is fit for assessment. In the past there has been a practice of waiting for a patient to be 'medically cleared' before referral to a mental health team. However, there is a big difference between a patient being 'fit for a psychiatric assessment', i.e. sober, not drowsy and ready to talk to someone and being 'fit for discharge', which can take several hours if blood tests and a period of observation is needed. If a patient has to wait to be fit for discharge before assessment by the mental health team, their length of stay in the ED will be much longer, and they may only have had a short conversation about their mental health, which was their main reason for attendance. The absolute ideal occurs when both teams work side by side, communicating well between them and putting the needs of the patient first. In the UK, the Royal College of Nursing, the College of Emergency Medicine, the College of Physicians and the Royal College of Psychiatrists have produced a joint position statement recommending this approach [5].

The practice of patients needing to be 'medically cleared' may be rooted in distrust between ED and mental health teams. At times ED clinicians have not got involved when someone presents with psychotic features, assuming that the problem is a psychiatric one. Conversely, mental health teams will be cautious about admitting a person who may have a medical cause for their psychotic symptoms. They also do not want to be in the position of having to decide whether a patient is medically fit for discharge. These fears and risks can only be managed by both ED and mental health teams working together.

6 Observation

Observations for patients who are considered to be at high risk of either self-harm, suicide or leaving before being assessed are another vital part of safety for mental health patients. Some EDs employ registered mental health nurses; others have registered adult nurses or health care assistants who may be allocated to observe a patient at risk. It is recommended that security staff should not be used in this role. Due to the unpredictability of some patients, this role can be quite challenging to perform, and training is required to help staff to observe them with safety in mind whilst simultaneously providing empathy and support.

Unless a therapeutic relationship is formed, continuous observation can make some patients feel more anxious or agitated. Intermittent observations can be therapeutic when that member of staff spends some time with the patient on arrival, checks in regularly with them to see if they need anything, keeps them updated and asks how they are feeling. This contributes towards excellent care and, contrary to some opinions, is very unlikely to make a person become a frequent attender.

7   Risk Assessment by ED Clinicians

Knowledge and skills needed to do an effective assessment of a patient presenting with a mental health problem are part of all Emergency Medicine curricula. Unfortunately, audit in the UK shows that not all clinicians document a risk assessment or a mental state examination [6], both of which are key for safe and excellent mental health emergency care. This may be because they feel that the mental health team are about to come and do this or that the patient may not want to go through this twice. However, by not asking anything about the patient's mental health, they may miss therapeutic opportunities to support and be empathetic. If the patient decides to leave before a member of the mental health team sees them, then they may not know how to safely respond to this.

The ED clinician's role is to do a brief risk assessment of self-harm, suicide and the risk of the patient leaving before assessment and treatment are complete. Their assessment may lead to a change in the requirement for continuous or intermittent observation. Most of a mental state examination is picked up by listening to the patient and observing their behaviour; however, to complete a mental state examination, the clinician should directly ask about suicidality and altered perceptions using the following criteria:

8   Mental State Examination

- Appearance
- Behaviour
- Mood
- Speech
- Thoughts including suicidality
- Perceptions/hallucinations
- Cognition
- Insight

ED clinicians should be familiar with the factors about a person and around a suicide attempt or self-harm episode which makes risks of further harm more likely. There are no validated risk assessment tools for use by ED or mental health professionals, and consequently NICE guidance warns against using such tools. Risk assessment of patients presenting to the ED is complex. Whilst of all completed suicides, 43% of people had been to ED the year before they took their life, only

25% had attended following self-harm. Of those that present to the ED with self-harm, 1% will die by suicide the following year, but identifying that 1% is very difficult. Approximately half of all suicides are in people that were regarded as having a low risk of suicide and of the people considered to be of high risk, the vast majority do not die. This is not to say that we should not attempt to assess risk, but the focus should be instead around safety planning—managing and reducing that risk with the patient and their family and friends.

9   Capacity Assessment by ED Clinicians

Assessment of a person's mental capacity for different decisions can be challenging. There are various pitfalls in assessing mental capacity. Many clinicians will be aware of the two-stage test for capacity in England outlined below (Fig. 1).

The following points help avoid common pitfalls in mental capacity assessments.

1. Mental capacity is time and decision specific.
   The phrase 'this patient lacks capacity' is inherently wrong. Instead, it could be said that 'currently this patient lacks the capacity *to decide to leave*'.
2. Capacity laws state that we should presume a person has capacity unless there is evidence to the contrary.
3. People are allowed to make what another person would think is an unwise decision.
4. Always assess risk at the same time as capacity. If a person is felt to have a high risk of further self-harm, then we would have to have a high level of certainty that the person has capacity to decide to leave. Very few patients who are acutely suicidal can be said to retain capacity to make this decision.
5. Assessing whether a person can understand, retain and communicate is usually relatively easy; it is whether that person can really weigh their decision which counts. If a person is very distressed, they may be unable to weigh a decision.
6. Opinions on whether a person lacks capacity may vary, and it is good practice to discuss difficult assessments with other professionals who are more experienced.

The MCA sets out a 2-stage test of capacity:

1) Does the person have an impairment of their mind or brain, whether as a result of an illness, or external factors such as alcohol or drug use?

2) Does the impairment mean the person is unable to make a specific decision when they need to? People can lack capacity to make decisions, but have capacity to make others. Mental capacity can also fluctuate with time – someone may lack capacity at one point in time, but may be able to make the same decision at a later point in time.

Where appropriate, people should be allowed the time to make a decision.

Fig. 1   2-stage assessment under the English Mental Capacity Act [7, 8]

10   Managing an Agitated Patient

Patients with agitation are unfortunately not uncommon in the ED. Patients may be intoxicated, frustrated, frightened or in pain, or they be psychotic or delirious so that their ideas of what is going on around them do not match with reality. Ideally, clinicians will spot when a patient is becoming anxious or agitated early on, find out why this is and intervene. Other times a patient arrives already in an agitated state, which is more challenging to de-escalate. The skill of de-escalation comes naturally to some professionals, but not to all. Workplaces should provide face-to-face training regularly. It can help to watch how colleagues attempt de-escalation and learn from what helped and what did not. A supportive debrief can be valuable after difficult situations. Below are some tips as to how to and how not to attempt to de-escalate.

Do

- If there is time, get some collateral history from ambulance and police before you start talking to the patient. Rapidly look up any background information you may have about the patient.
- Be calm and introduce yourself; find out the name they like to be called.
- Present yourself with nonthreatening body language and tone of voice.
- Starting with a 'say what you know or see' empathic statement may help. 'It looks like you are quite frustrated just now' or 'It sounds as though you have had a difficult night tonight'.
- Offer to help. 'We are here to help'.
- Ask relevant questions—Did they choose to come to hospital? Who called for help? Are they in pain? Do they understand how they came to be in hospital? What would help them just now? Would an oral anxiolytic medicine help?
- If security or police are involved, work with them to try to step down any restraint or presence as soon as it is safe.
- Emphasise safety for the patient and those around them.
- Stick to firm boundaries.

Don't

- Tell a person to calm down!! This is rarely effective.
- Get too close or get between them and your exit.
- Threaten or bargain with them.
- Chastise them for being agitated.

Body-worn cameras can be a helpful addition when faced with a patient who is agitated. The patient should be told that the camera is being switched on and recording started. Discretion is needed as to when this is useful; however, it can also be a learning tool for staff after the event.

If de-escalation fails and the person is a risk to themselves, then the person may need restraint in order to keep them safe. Any restraint should be proportionate to the risk posed and be the minimum force for the minimum length of time. NICE [9] guidance states that if restraint is needed for more than 10 min, then rapid tranquilisation should be considered. Rapid tranquilisation usually consists of a dose of benzodiazepine (e.g. lorazepam or midazolam) or a combination of promethazine and haloperidol, initially offered orally, or if this is not accepted, IM or occasionally IV. Some centres use droperidol or olanzapine. The patient should be closely monitored after any sedative medication. Both restraint and rapid tranquilisation should be led by an experienced clinician who should stay present as far as is possible. There should be a goal in mind, e.g. to facilitate further assessment or to allow time for drugs to wear off.

11 Attitudes and Training

'It must be a full moon'.
'Not again'.
'It is just attention seeking…'.

Prejudiced and seemingly unsympathetic opinions may be heard in EDs and can unfortunately become contagious. Attitudes of ED staff to patients with mental health problems are complex. A few just do not understand the abstract nature of mental ill-health and do not know how to speak to people who display altered thinking processes. In the absence of training in communication techniques, this is understandable. Some are frustrated with a lack of community mental health services and feel that patients should be able to access help elsewhere. They may feel poorly prepared and under-resourced to provide care, which can spill out into frustration towards patients.

These attitudes can be influenced in various ways, such as through good role modelling from leaders, training from experts and providing resources to care. All professionals should be encouraged to actively challenge unhelpful comments and behaviour amongst their colleagues. One of the most effective ways to change attitudes is to allow staff to understand how an individual came to be in the situation that they are in. This can particularly be helpful with patients that attend frequently. A concise management plan made with a patient, which outlines previous events, describes what their triggers may be for a crisis and what helps and hinders them can be useful to understand different behaviours.

12 A Safe and Calm Environment

Emergency departments are predominantly designed for patients with physical illness. The environment can be busy and overstimulating; it lacks quiet spaces and has physical risks such as potential points for ligatures. Most departments have safe rooms for psychiatric assessment, with two doors, no ligature points, and with the right furniture/fittings which cannot become a weapon. However, departments struggle to provide safe, quiet and calm environments for patients whilst they are being treated or are waiting for assessment.

Where possible, quiet safe spaces where patients can be observed and treated should be added to our departments. A glass door which shuts out noise but allows a patient to be observed may help some. Departments need to assess for potential ligature points and other potentials for harm. Additionally, there may be challenges of not having sufficient staffing to provide adequate care and observation of patients. Mental health needs to be high on an organisation's priorities and risk registers in order to have sufficient staff with mental health training to care for patients.

13   Legal Frameworks Within the ED

Legal frameworks for patients with severe mental illness vary in different countries. ED staff should be familiar with their own legislation, when to apply and how to manage documentation of use of this legislation. Policies for each geographical system are required, and governance to ensure compliance with policies and legal requirements should be in place. Remember that having to treat a person against their will can be very stressful, so good explanation, support and reassurance are needed.

14   Frequent Attendance to the ED

Patients who attend EDs frequently with mental health problems can be challenging to manage. They may have a combination of mental health, social stressors and drug and alcohol problems. For some, the ED may be a safe place that gets them through a crisis and even keeps them alive. For others, they do not want to come but are brought by family, friends or police.

Ways of managing frequent attendances include:

1. Information sharing—between mental health, primary care, police and ambulance services—is helpful to manage risk and improve consistency of care. This may take the form of a regular multidisciplinary team meeting.
2. Case management—involves working with the individual to help address their needs, e.g. housing, accessing addiction services, finances, etc.
3. Shared management plans—these are best co-produced with the individual where possible. They should involve background information on that person, what their triggers are, what helps and hinders when they come to ED and suggestions for how to manage their crisis.

The impact of these three interventions on attendances to ED is modest. Case management has the best evidence base, yielding moderate cost savings but with variable reduction in attendances [10]. Shared management plans do not reduce attendances [11], but they improve staff confidence in managing patients and almost certainly improve safety.

15   Conclusion

Emergency departments still have a way to go to provide kind, safe and excellent care for patients experiencing mental health crisis. It is helpful to think about safety at every stage of a patient's journey through the ED, to challenge poor care and to prioritise training for all staff groups to improve knowledge and skills.

Learning Points

- Attitudes to mental health are still a problem. ED care for patients can be improved by listening to patients' experiences and trying to see things from their point of view.
- Sometimes the ED is just there to get someone through a crisis in the same way we get people through diabetic or asthmatic crises. Many lives may be saved this way.
- Mental health care in ED is best delivered as a team with ED nursing, clinical and liaison psychiatry staff working closely together.

References

1. Baracaia S, McNulty D, Baldwin S, Mytton J, Evison F, Raine R, Giacco D, Hutchings A, Barratt H. Mental health in hospital emergency department: a cross-sectional analysis of attendances in England 2013/14. Emerg Med J. 2020:744–51.
2. NHS Digital. Hospital episode statistics; 2020. Available at: https://digital.nhs.uk/data-and-information/data-tools-and-services/data-services/hospital-episode-statistics.   Accessed March 2021.
3. Australian Government Department of Health. Mental health triage tool. 2013. https://www1.health.gov.au/internet/publications/publishing.nsf/Content/triageqrg~triageqrg-mh. Accessed July 2021.
4. Broadbent M, Jarman H, Berk M. Emergency department mental health triage scales improve outcomes. J Eval Clin Pract. 2004;10(1):57–62.
5. Royal College of Psychiatrists, Royal College of Nurses, Royal College of Emergency Medicine, & Royal College of Physicians. Side by side: a UK-wide consensus statement on working together to help patients with mental health needs in acute hospitals. https://www.rcpsych.ac.uk/docs/default-source/members/faculties/liaison-psychiatry/liaison-sidebyside.pdf. Published by RCPsych, London; 2020.
6. Royal College of Emergency Medicine (RCEM). Mental health (self-harm) National quality improvement project report. National Report 2019/20. London: RCEM; 2021. https://www.rcem.ac.uk//docs/RCEM%20Mental%20Health%20national%20report%20FINAL.pdf
7. Mental Capacity Act. Crown copyright: London; 2005. https://www.legislation.gov.uk/ukpga/2005/9/contents. Accessed 20th January 2022.
8. NHS. Mental capacity act. 2005. https://www.nhs.uk/conditions/social-care-and-support-guide/making-decisions-for-someone-else/mental-capacity-act/
9. NICE. Violence and aggression: short-term management in mental health, health and community settings. NICE guideline [NG10] Published: 28 May 2015. NICE guidance. 2015. https://www.nice.org.uk/guidance/ng10restraint
10. Soril LJJ, Leggett LE, Lorenzetti DL, Noseworthy TW, Clement FM. Reducing frequent visits to the emergency department: a systematic review of interventions. PLoS One. 2015;10(4):e0123660. https://doi.org/10.1371/journal.pone.0123660.
11. Spillane LL, Lumb EW, Cobaugh DJ, Wilcox SR, Clark JS, Schneider SM. Frequent users of the emergency department: can we intervene? Acad Emerg Med. 1997;4:574–80. pmid: 9189190

Mental Health Liaison Team

Kieran Quirke

1   Introduction

Several years ago, at the annual Royal College of Psychiatrist's PLAN Conference, Dr. Peter Aitken—then faculty chair and giving that year's keynote speech—began his talk with a slide which featured a range of images of what might only be described as everyday stress and strain. What is it we see coming through the doors of emergency departments (EDs) up and down the country, every day of the week? The answer he gave—as simple as it sounds—'all life'. This is a truth which will ring clearly with every liaison nurse, doctor and allied clinician working in the field, all of whom will recognise the times they have needed to act not just as a healthcare professional but as counsellor, housing advisor or drug worker and the times they have had to address legal problems, employment difficulties and relationship break-ups. It reflects the vast range of presentations which a liaison clinician might encounter in the course of a shift, from a florid psychosis to a set of lost keys. The unique positioning of the ED, with 24-h access to immediate care and support creates an environment where those problems—'all life'—converge.

Liaison psychiatry is a subspeciality of clinical psychiatry concerned with the assessment and treatment of patients within the general hospital setting. It sits at the interface between physical and mental health and is essentially an answer to the mind-body dualism that has dominated medicine for centuries and that patients must be approached with a holistic, collaborative mindset to redress not only the shocking health inequalities and early mortality experienced by a significant proportion of patients with severe and enduring mental illness but the vast unmet needs of patients who develop a mental health problem consequent of a physical illness.

K. Quirke (✉)
Associate Director of Nursing for Mental Health, King's College Hospital NHS Foundation Trust, London, UK
e-mail: kieran.quirke@nhs.net

© The Author(s), under exclusive license to Springer Nature Switzerland AG 2023
T. Scott (ed.), *Mental Health: Intervention Skills for the Emergency Services*,
https://doi.org/10.1007/978-3-031-20347-3_6

The role of the ED in the assessment and care of those in mental health crisis is a contentious issue and has attracted increased focus during the COVID-19 pandemic, as services and resources have been subject to inevitable shift and change. The often frenetic and noisy environment of the ED floor is far from suited to the patient group, and there have been numerous stories in recent years of long delays and wait times, alongside resource shortages in some areas of the country which has added to suggestions that emergency mental health care is better placed elsewhere. While there is certainly an argument to be had for creating alternative avenues of help, particularly for patients already under community teams requiring out-of-hours support, patients will continue to present to EDs in crisis—and rightly so. The concept of 'parity of esteem', enshrined in the NHS' Five Year Forward View for Mental Health [1], cannot be achieved if we are to return to operating in silos—any environmental challenge can be overcome with dedicated, creative thinking to ensure facilities are not simply adequate but designed from the ground up with the specific needs of this patient group in mind.

Although there is relatively limited research available, the total number of global mental health presentations to EDs has been estimated to be around 4% [2]. This is mirrored in the UK, where a similar proportion has been estimated at between 4 and 5% [3, 4]. Indeed, UK national data shows attendances are rising year on year, increasing by 133% between 2009 and 2018 [5].

The ED at London's King's College Hospital, a 950-bed general hospital and major trauma centre, addresses the needs of around 120,000 patients a year, with approximately 350 patients attending each day. The Liaison Team sees around 3–4% of these. Patients primarily come from Lambeth and Southwark; both boroughs are socially disparate and sit in the bottom quartile of the most deprived local authorities in England causing a significant effect on multimorbidities [6, 7], and both boroughs have historically experienced high mental health need.

Appendix 1 contains a range of charts (Figs. 1, 2, 3, 4, 5, 6, 7, and 8) which show the King's team data over a 3-month period between November 2020 and January 2021 (this choice of months may appear slightly arbitrary but was selected as the figures provided a very typical representation of the Liaison Team's activity, with the months occurring as they did with a lower number of COVID-19-related restrictions. At other times in 2020 restrictions had caused varying impact on attendance). The team typically will receive around 300 referrals from the department per calendar month (Fig. 1), but this can vary widely dependent on the time of year, with some months recording closer to 400. Presentations are broadly evenly split between male and female, with a lightly higher percentage of males attending (Fig. 2). The majority 53% of patients referred fall between the ages of 25 and 49, with the remainder again evenly split between the younger and older age groups outside this category and a small percentage of over 65 s (Fig. 3). Figure 4 shows times of presentations across the 24-h period; the Liaison team—mirroring the ED—generally sees periods of higher acuity from midday onwards, reaching a peak between early afternoon and late evening.

2 King's Liaison Psychiatry Service

The department of Psychological Medicine at King's houses a number of sub-teams and work streams including psychology, alcohol care and outpatients across various medical specialities. The Liaison team itself comprises three sub-teams—older adults, inpatients and the ED. While there is some sharing of resources across the three sub-teams, with the Liaison consultants providing clinical oversight to the ED and acting (along with the team's rotational speciality trainees) as second opinion for Mental Health Act assessments, the teams operate mostly on a separate basis and the ED team is nurse-led.

The team structure falls somewhere between the enhanced and comprehensive Core24 service models developed in 2014 [8]. Under a Clinical Service Lead with managerial responsibility for the entire liaison psychiatry department, the ED sub-team comprises a Band 7 team leader overseeing a further six Band 7 senior PLNs. The team has funding for a further 11 NHS Band 6 PLNs and currently also has 2 NHS Band 5 RMNs, who are employed by the mental health trust but part funded by the acute trust and a dedicated administrator.

The size of the psychological medicine department has meant locating all three sub-teams in a central space has not been possible to date, but despite the disadvantages this separation brings, there is one particular positive for the PLN team; it allows the PLNs to occupy an office space within the ED footprint, providing greater integration and presence within the ED team. The relationship between the liaison service and the wider ED team is pivotal and co-location, and the visibility of the nurses within the department is integral to this. This is aided further by participation in training initiatives, and the PLN team facilitates a mental health awareness training session for the ED team several times a year, participates in the Capital Nurse training scheme and delivers periodic 'bite-size' training sessions on selected topics such as Section 136 at varying intervals.

3 Legislative and Ethical Issues

Liaison nurses are required to have a sound understanding of both the Mental Capacity Act [9] and the Mental Health Act [10] in order to be able to carry out their roles effectively. The ED will see many cases, from simple to highly complex, of patients lacking capacity. While not a primary function of the team, the skillset of the liaison nurse positions them as a useful resource to assist the ED team in the assessment of capacity elsewhere in the department.

Decisions around capacity are a pivotal part of any dynamic risk assessment and require careful consideration, though, for the PLNs, this conversely often needs to happen at speed. The busy and fast-paced ED is not the ideal environment for reaching these sorts of quick decisions, and the PLNs need to be able to read situations and act in a manner that maintains safety without causing unnecessary restriction. PLNs frequently receive calls asking for immediate assistance because a patient is demanding to leave, for example, raising an alarm and summoning security to assist might be vital in one scenario, where the risk is evident, but heavy handed in another with the consequent danger of restricting liberty without cause. Ultimately, the PLNs must be able to justify their clinical decisions in the best interests of the patient. Navigating this difficult legal tightrope skilfully comes with clinical experience in crisis mental health care and is one of the reasons why PLN work is not suited to newly qualified nurses.

The well documented mental health bed crisis across the UK is no different at King's than anywhere else; there is insufficient continuous inpatient capacity to meet demand, and patients are frequently required to wait considerable periods of time before either formal or informal admission to inpatient beds. In the case of formal admission, no identifiable bed can mean a period of many hours waiting in the ED midway through an incomplete Mental Health Act assessment. Until the Approved Mental Health Professional signs the paperwork and while awaiting transfer, the patient becomes 'liable to be detained' and detention can only be legally justified using the Mental Capacity Act.

The *Sessay* vs *South London and Maudsley NHS Trust* 2011 judgement looms somewhat largely over all liaison services in the above regard. This case involved a woman who was brought by police from her home to the Maudsley Hospital's Section 136 facility, the Emergency Clinic. The police took her there using the framework of the Mental Capacity Act but even prior to the court judgement accepted that, outside of using Sections 135 and 136, they had no legal right to do so. *Sessay* also had to wait in the Emergency Clinic for 13 h from arrival to admission and made a case that she had unlawfully been deprived of her liberty during this time. The trust presented the argument that the Mental Health Act did not provide for all circumstances in which there might be delays in processing admission, but the court rejected this, pointing towards provisions in Section 4 and elsewhere which were already in place to address such delays [11].

Section 4 allows for the emergency detention of a person using only a single medical recommendation and either an AMHP or nearest relative's opinion, in situations where waiting to organise a full Mental Health Act assessment would cause 'undue delay'. This is of little use to liaison nurses working in metropolitan areas where similar delays in the ED are typically the result of bed availability rather than access to sufficient AMHPs and s12 doctors. However, *Sessay* contained a very important additional point, which remains very relevant to ED liaison psychiatry. The court wrote that every case would need to be decided on its own merits, but that so long as it was clear there was no 'undue delay' in the processing of an application under the MHA, a court would be unlikely to rule that deprivation of liberty had occurred. Given the severity and urgency of Mental Health Act assessments in the ED, so long as it is supported by thorough documentation containing adequate and appropriate capacity assessment and chronological narrative evidencing the steps the liaison nurses have taken to move the assessment on, e.g. calls to bed managers or AMHP teams, it is unlikely the court will find fault.

King's, like most liaison services, relies heavily on support from the local trust security team. In the absence of sufficient RMN capacity to meet demand at times, often due to a lack of available staff rather than anything else, security is often relied upon to provide assistance in ensuring high-risk patients do not abscond from the department. The King's security team provide an excellent service despite considerable demands on their limited resources, and the good working relationship we continue to maintain with them hinges on clear and continuous communication of risk, capacity and the legal frameworks being used to prevent someone requiring detention under the MHA from leaving.

At the current time, the King's Liaison Team has the use of two high-risk assessment rooms in the Majors area of the ED, along with two lower risk rooms in the Urgent Care Centre. While there are not specific or formal criteria for allocation, the decision regarding where to place people is typically collaborative between the ED team and liaison and will focus on individual presentations along with absconsion, violence or self-harm risks. The high-risk rooms are designed to meet PLAN standards [12] and are ligature-proof and have seclusion-type furniture and two-way opening doors at either end. The rooms are not perfect though spacious enough to accommodate four people, they are sparsely decorated and given that some patients will spend a number of hours within them, work is already underway to consider ways in which décor can be improved additional comfort and stimulation without compromising safety.

At King's, the location of the rooms has previously posed challenges in relation to maintaining privacy and dignity for the patients using them. The rooms are situated opposite a row of chairs used to seat patients admitted to the department but waiting for the next step of their journey through the ED. With the risk of having to accompany a floridly unwell person into the rooms past an 'audience', an additional entrance was placed at the side of the rooms avoiding this area, along with a small foyer and ligature-proof toilet, giving patients access to facilities without having to walk through the busy department.

4 Referral Routes

The Liaison Team is integrated into the wider ED service, and as such, all referrals are via the usual route into the ED; patients will present either by themselves (sometimes accompanied by another health professional or community worker) or might arrive by ambulance or with police. The team does not accept direct referrals from outside of the department, though encourages strong lines of communication with any external teams intending to send patients to the ED for mental health assessment. This is not with the intention of discouraging that course of action (though sometimes it can be helpful to consider alternative sources of support and divert away from the ED when it is clear a lower level of support might be more appropriate). Crucially, this allows for an exchange of collateral information as quickly as possible, particularly given the community worker is likely to hold a much more intimate knowledge of the patient and their insight can only improve the quality and safety of the subsequent PLN assessment.

The origins of referrals can be varied and come from many different sources. Housing departments, hostels, education providers, General Practitioner surgeries, crisis lines; the list is endless, and all can and do advise patients to attend the ED if concerned. A shortage of other services offering immediate crisis assessment has meant that community mental health teams and home treatment teams may bring patients to the department, often to wait for admission in the absence of a safe alternative.

On arrival, patients are triaged by the ED nursing team, who use a simple proprietary colour-coded assessment tool to categorise and identify immediate risk. The tool allows for a quick identification of patients who might benefit from the utilisation of immediate resources, such as one to one nursing observations, or the involvement of the hospital security team. The triage nurse will call through and speak with the senior PLN on shift and provide a basic handover, and then the senior PLN is tasked with quickly screening the patient to again ascertain risk, to assess why the patient has come and what intervention they are likely to require. On occasion, if it can be achieved quickly and safely, the senior PLN may reach the conclusion the patient does not require full assessment and instead can be signposted to an alternative community resource for support. However, in most instances the senior PLN will ask one of the NHS Band 6 PLNs to see the patient and carry out a full biopsychosocial assessment; the senior PLN will provide oversight and senior clinical opinion if required, while functioning as the central voice of the liaison team, the co-ordinator and manager of flow through the department for the duration of their shift.

The evidence-based treatment pathway [13] set a number of targets liaison teams were expected to achieve. The first was response time, with a target that every emergency referral would be seen within 1 h. The dynamic nature of the senior PLN NHS Band 7 role, with quick screening and oversight of flow through the department, allows for this to happen in almost all instances, and the King's team is able to see on average between 94 and 96% of ED patients within this time frame (Fig. 5). A second target was that all patients should have been assessed and have a discharge plan in place within 4 h. While the King's liaison team achieves this in almost all cases, it does not prevent patients from staying longer than this in the department, at times for medical reasons, at others due to the complexity of the presenting case and at others due to issues with flow. A national bed crisis in mental health means that despite best efforts to accommodate inpatient admissions in as timely a manner as possible, patients will still frequently experience long delays in waiting for bed allocation. Figure 5 shows both the median and mean wait times at King's; while the median sits at around the 3-h mark, the mean is significantly higher falling between 6.5 and 8 h, due to the small number of patients whose wait for a bed stretches beyond the 12-h breach mark.

Referrals within the ED can come from any clinician currently working on that shift and at any stage in the patient's journey through the department. The intent of the liaison service is to work *in parallel* with the ED team in every case, to prevent wasted hours and ensure patient flow as efficiently as possible, a benefit to both patient and the organisation. There are obviously times when this is neither possible nor appropriate, for example, a patient with a very acute onset of psychotic symptoms and no previous history would benefit from a focus on their medical status in the first instance. It will be difficult, if not impossible, to reach a conclusion from a psychiatric perspective about what is happening for them without this; however, in many cases, parallel working is appropriate and not only saves time but can also enhance patient assessment and experience, as by its nature it means closer and more collaborative and integrated working between mental health and acute trust staff. The enemy of parallel working is the much-misappropriated term 'medical clearance', which has on many occasions needlessly delayed psychiatric assessment for no clear justification or rationale.

King's has developed a unique approach to the management of acutely disturbed or violent patients in the ED, known as 'Code 10' (Appendix 2). Created in collaboration between the ED medical team and liaison service, Code 10 provides a system for an immediate multidisciplinary review of any patient meeting the criteria, with the aim of implementing safe, fast and efficient management plans to stabilise the patient and in turn reduce the risk of staff assault. Code 10 can be triggered by any member of staff through a call to switchboard and subsequently communicated immediately to a number of key staff carrying bleeps—the consultant and senior ED nurse on shift, the senior liaison PLN, the liaison duty core trainee and the security team shift leader. Furthermore, local police and ambulance services have been included in the process and can call in advance if bringing a patient to the department who meets the criteria, ensuring a team can be ready to meet them on arrival and a full multidisciplinary team handover and management plan can be quickly put in place.

Code 10 is utilised in all cases where a patient is brought to the ED under Section 136. The introduction of London's Section 136 Pathway [14] helped address long-standing arguments across the country as to whether an ED constituted a 'place of safety' in the context of the Mental Health Act. The answer is that it does though this assumption is tempered by an acknowledgement that the ED environment held particular challenges when compared to dedicated s136 suites and health-based places of safety, and the document advises both a collaborative approach between the ED and the police in managing the patient along with authorisation to use s136 in the department itself. South London and Maudsley NHS Foundation Trust operates a Centralised Place of Safety covering all four boroughs of the Trust geography, and the expectation is that s136 patients are taken there in the first instance. There are times however when bed space is not available, and the ED will be the next port of call for police, so the pathway equally makes clear the expectations and duties of liaison services in ensuring patients are not left waiting hours for assessment. The liaison team at King's, in collaboration with acute staff, the police and the local Centralised Place of Safety team based at the Maudsley Hospital has developed a specific s136 pathway document to make roles and responsibilities clear (Appendix 3). The flowchart centres on quick acceptance to the department, early assessment and clear communication between all teams involved.

5   Presentations

The types of presentations seen within the service are many and varied. Most liaison clinicians could quite probably fill a book with the more unusual stories they have encountered during their work. Exactly what constitutes a crisis is relative to all of us, and this is reflected in the range of needs that cross the ED threshold; many patients will attend with issues stemming from difficulties in their social circumstances or other areas of their personal lives. More will present with a number of problems which might be difficult to distil down into a single neat field of data. This has created challenges in piecing together an accurate picture of attendance reasons that truly reflect the core circumstances of the patients using the service.

Figure 6 shows the primary attendance reasons for patients referred to the team between November 2020 and January 2021. Suicidal ideation and acts of deliberate self-harm make up over half of all patients referred to the service, closely followed by psychotic symptoms or odd behaviour. Self-harm statistics for EDs have been considered unreliable in the past, with severe under-reporting of official data [15], but 220,000 annual episodes across the UK have been estimated [16]. The data for King's broadly fits in line with this estimate proportional to overall attendances. Figure 7 provides a more detailed view of self-harm presentations; overdose is by far the most common presenting method of self-harm, accounting for nearly two thirds of all DSH attendances. Other particularly violent forms of self-harm, e.g. jumping from a height, which accounts for 7% of attendances, reflect King's status as a major trauma centre covering a large part of the southeast; as a consequence, the department sees a large number of traumatic injuries each year resulting from incidents of self-harm.

6   Interventions and Support Paths

The majority of patients referred to the service will receive a full biopsychosocial assessment, a holistic view of their presentation incorporating attention to physical, psychological and social needs before a formulation is reached and a discharge plan created. Brief interventions based on solution-focussed or cognitive-behavioural principles may be offered dependent on circumstance and the clinician's experience and skill.

Figure 8 details patient discharge destinations for the period between November 2020 and January 2021. A small number of patients are admitted to mental health inpatient wards, with a slightly higher percentage (9%) detained formally under the Mental Health Act, compared to voluntary or informal admissions (7%). The majority of discharged patients go to community mental health teams for follow-up, and the liaison team has 'trusted assessor' status with these teams, bypassing single point of access or other preliminary triage stages that might otherwise exist. The 8% of patients discharged to GP and voluntary services is likely to be an underestimate arising again from the difficulties in collating data where there may be multiple outcomes; many patients are provided with the details of local voluntary services on exit from the department, even if not directly referred. The liaison team has strong links with a range of these, such as Solidarity in a Crisis, a peer support programme specifically for local EDs of brief community engagement and support; similarly, the Evening Sanctuary offers an evening support service for Lambeth residents, and the Listening Place is a free and responsive support service for patients from across London experiencing suicidal ideation. In the case of the Listening Place, the King's liaison team quickly became one of its largest sources of referrals following its creation in 2015, leading the acute trust to build on this relationship and offer space within the hospital for the service to run satellite clinics, an excellent example of collaborative working between the statutory and nonstatutory sectors.

The problem of frequent attenders more commonly defined as patients who attend the ED five or more times in a year [17] is one experienced not just by liaison teams and EDs within the UK but throughout the world. Frequent attenders make up a sizeable proportion of all ED attendees; one recent study estimated as many as one in ten patients met the criteria of a frequent attender and accounted for 25% of total ED presentations [18]. While not all of these patients attend for mental health reasons, there is often a psychological component. For those whose frequent attendances directly relate to mental health issues, the liaison service will work collaboratively with their community teams to try and reduce frequency, providing a voice at community MDTs and producing co-operative management plans.

The acute trust holds a monthly frequent attenders meeting at which ED and liaison team staff, hospital social workers and London Ambulance Service NHS Trust representation will review a list of patients who have attended four or more times in the previous month. This provides an opportunity for co-ordinating a departmental response including the involvement of other agencies in the patient's care and the development of bespoke care plans and strategies to try and move the patient away from their dependency on the ED to other more helpful sources of support.

7   Evaluations and the Future of the Service

The service receives 3-yearly evaluation and accreditation from the Royal College of Psychiatrist's PLAN team. This involves an evaluation set against the PLAN standards [12], a comprehensive set of expected criteria which all liaison services are expected to meet, from the safety and specification of assessment rooms to documentation to patient feedback mechanisms. The PLAN standards are mapped to the Health and Social Care Act 2008 (Regulated Activities) Regulations [19], and the assessment of the service is conducted by a group of independent professional liaison and service user representatives.

In March 2020, in response to the declaration of the COVID-19 pandemic, a letter was sent from Claire Murdoch, Head of Mental Health for NHS England to the chief executives of all UK Mental Health Trusts. The letter made a request not only to bolster remote support services such as crisis helplines but also to consider alternative arrangements that might be taken to see patients in mental health crisis away from the ED. The intention was to relieve as much pressure from the acute trusts as possible in the expectation of a surge of respiratory cases. Most mental health trusts immediately began developing and opening crisis diversion units. In the case of South London and Maudsley NHS Foundation Trust, a new service, the Crisis Assessment Unit (CAU) was opened on the site of the Maudsley's outpatients building. The CAU was a five-bedded alternative to the ED, staffed jointly by liaison nurses and doctors from King's and St Thomas' Hospital. This was a challenge in itself given that a reduced liaison service would still need to be present at both sites throughout, and while numbers initially dropped by around a third in the first lockdown of April 2020, by May they had started to increase to levels above what would usually be expected.

In essence, CAU was expected to run as a mirror image of the liaison team in the ED. Patients would not self-present and would still attend the general hospital, but the NHS Band 7 on site would very quickly screen for suitability against a set of exclusion criteria and, if appropriate, immediately transfer the patient to the diversion space. Putting aside the rationale for the unit and the atypical circumstances of a global pandemic, the existence of CAU and other diversion spaces across the UK provided a useful experiment for future service models of liaison within EDs. The negatives were obvious immediately, e.g. a return to operational silos and a potential major blow to the concept of parity of esteem, something hard-fought in EDs up and down the country over many years by liaison colleagues. Anecdotal reports reinforced this, suggesting the unwelcome return of unhelpful and negative views towards mental health patients among a small minority of ED staff. Legal issues, such as the transfer of patients lacking capacity and safety concerned the danger of patients being transferred without adequate medical triage, were also evident. In addition, the creation of the service underlined how few patients met the criteria for transfer to the service and just how many required the dual model of physical and mental health care provided for in the ED.

There was at least one undeniable positive however. The ability to create an environment much calmer and more appropriate to the needs of mental health patients than an ED would ever be able to provide, regardless of how much time and effort might be spent on improving the décor and facilities of individual assessment rooms, a relative calm that could only be achieved with some element of distance from the highly charged milieu of the ED. A hybrid model in the shape of a mental health Clinical Decision Unit co-located on the acute trust site (ideally next to or attached to the respective ED) might therefore prove the way forwards for future liaison services, a service able to provide the calm and therapeutic environment often lacking in EDs and often the source of criticism of mental health care in the ED in general, but one which continues to operate as a joint, not siloed venture and ideally, with an integrated, co-staffing model.

8   Conclusion

Over 3500 referrals are typically made to the nurse-led liaison psychiatry service at King's College Hospital every year, with the majority coming from the local boroughs of Lambeth and Southwark, areas with high levels of deprivation and mental health need. Presentations to the service are varied, but most common referral reasons are due to suicidal ideation, psychotic symptoms or deliberate self-harm. The hospital's status as a major trauma centre means that the team encounters a significant number of cases of serious and violent self-harm causing traumatic injuries every year. Over the two decades the team has been in operation, it has become increasingly integrated into the fabric of the acute hospital, and the temporary split to staff and running a diversion space off-site during the earlier stages of the pandemic underlined the need for a 24-h ED-based service. That experimental period has also brought the future of the service into focus, and moving forwards may well provide answers as to how the service can remain a part of the ED and continue to provide high-quality patient care but do so in an environment specifically created with the needs and requirements of the patient group in mind.

Learning Points
- Identify the main five patient presentations which required mental health liaison within your department. What is the referral process?
- Outline salient mental health legislation to protect the interests of mental health patients when attending the emergency department.
- Consider the experience of people who attend the emergency department in mental health crisis. What are their immediate needs?

Appendix 1 King's Liaison Data, November 2020: January 2021

Fig. 1 Referral numbers by month

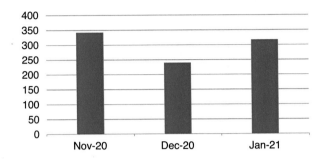

Fig. 2 Presentations by gender

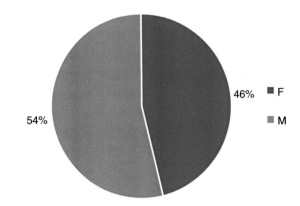

Fig. 3 Presentations by age group

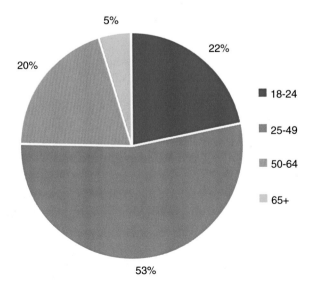

Fig. 4 Presentations by time

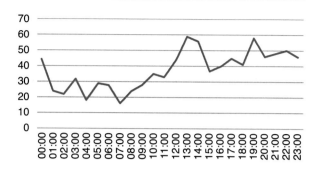

Fig. 5 Response rate, median and mean total wait times

Month	Seen within 1 hour	Median total wait time	Mean total wait time
November 2020	97%	3 hours 6 minutes	7 hours 46 minutes
December 2020	96%	4 hours 13 minutes	7 hours 52 minutes
January 2021	94%	3 hours 37 minutes	6 hours 28 minutes

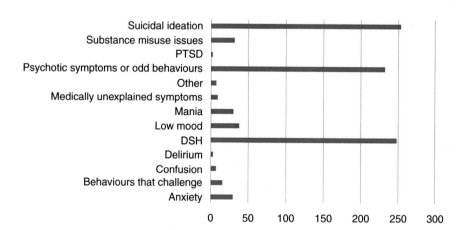

Fig. 6 Attendance reasons

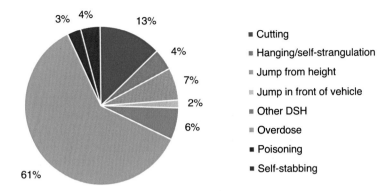

Fig. 7 Self-harm by type

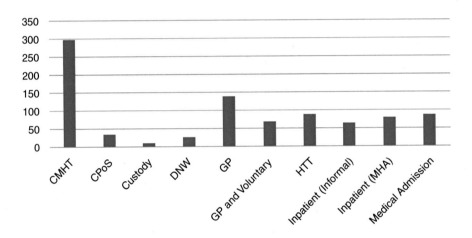

Fig. 8 Discharge destinations

Appendix 2 Code 10 Pathway

CODE 10 PATHWAY
Dr J Butier/ Dr O Mizzi
KCH ED MH Steering Group
March 2016

"CODE 10"
KCH Emergency Department - Denmark Hill

"CODE 10" activated
- Tannoy & can 2222
- Notify Security X34567

"CODE 10" team assemble
- ED senior Doctor
- ED NIC & ED nurse
- MH team (PIANP/PLN & Doctor)
- KCH Security / KCH Police Liaison (if available)

Handover from Police / LAS / ED staff
- Brief history of events
- Under MH section?
- Under arrest?
- Mental capacity concerns
- Medical concerns

Decide initial management plan / priorities
- Security / safety
- Rapid tranquillisation?
- Medical Investigation / treatment?
- MH assessment

Concurrent medical and MH assessment where possible

Early plan for disposition from the ED
- Admission to KCH - establish if security / RMN needed on ward
- Formal MH assessment pathway in ED
- Transfer to S136 suite with police
- Transfer to police custody

Appendix 3: Section 136 Pathway

Section 136 Flowchart

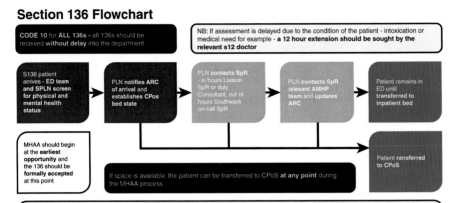

Draft v0.5 03/11/20

References

1. NHS England. NHS five year forward view. United Kingdom: NHS England; 2014.
2. Barratt H, Rojas-García A, Clarke K, Moore A, Whittington C, Stockton S, Thomas J, Pilling S, Raine R. Epidemiology of mental health attendances at emergency departments: systematic review and meta-analysis. PLoS One. 2016;11(4):e0154449.
3. Baracaia S, McNulty D, Baldwin S, Mytton J, Evison F, Raine R, Giacco D, Hutchings A, Barratt H. Mental health in hospital emergency departments: cross-sectional analysis of attendances in England 2013/2014. Emerg Med J. 2020;37(12):744–51.
4. Healthcare Safety Investigation Branch. Investigation into the provision of mental health care to patients presenting at the emergency department [Online]. 2018. Available at: https://www.hsib.org.uk/documents/65/HSIB_Provision_of_Mental_Health_in_ED_I2017006_Full_report.pdf
5. NHS Digital. Hospital accident and emergency activity, 2017-18. [Online] NHS Digital. 2018. Available at: https://digital.nhs.uk/data-and-information/publications/statistical/hospital-accident%2D%2Demergency-activity/2017-18
6. Lambeth Together. Latest research from Lambeth DataNet–Lambeth together [Online]. 2019. lambethtogether.net. Available at: https://lambethtogether.net/latest-research-from-lambeth-datanet/
7. Southwark Public Health Division. Indices of deprivation 2019 JSNA factsheet: Southwark's Joint strategic needs assessment [Online]. 2019. Available at: https://www.southwark.gov.uk/assets/attach/11987/JSNA-2019-Indices-of-Deprivation-2019.pdf
8. Aitken P, Robens S, Emmens T (eds). Developing models for liaison psychiatry services–guidance [Online]. 2014. Available at: https://mentalhealthpartnerships.com/wp-content/uploads/sites/3/3-developing-models-for-liaison-psychiatry-services.pdf
9. Mental Capacity Act. Crown copyright. London. 2005. https://www.legislation.gov.uk/ukpga/2005/9/contents. Accessed 20 Jan 2022.

10. Mental Health Act. Crown copyright. London. 2007. https://www.legislation.gov.uk/ukpga/2007/12/contents. Accessed 31 Mar 2022.
11. 39 Essex Chambers. R (Sessay) v SLAM & Commissioner of the police for the metropolis|39 Essex Chambers|Barristers' Chambers [Online]. (2011. Available at: https://www.39essex.com/cop_cases/r-sessay-v-slam-and-commissioner-of-the-police-for-the-metropolis/
12. Psychiatric Liaison Accreditation Network. Psychiatric liaison accreditation network (PLAN) quality standards for liaison psychiatry services, Sixth Edition [Online]. 2020. Available at: https://www.rcpsych.ac.uk/docs/default-source/improving-care/ccqi/quality-networks/psychi-atric-liaison-services-plan/quality-standards-for-liaison-psychiatry-services%2D%2D-sixth-edition-20209b6be47cb0f249f697850e1222d6b6e1.pdf?sfvrsn=1ddd53f2_0
13. NHS England, NICE, NCCMH. Achieving better access to 24/7 urgent and emergency mental health care–Part 2: implementing the evidence-based treatment pathway for urgent and emergency liaison mental health services for adults and older adults–guidance [Online]. 2016. Available at: https://www.england.nhs.uk/wp-content/uploads/2016/11/lmhs-guidance.pdf
14. Healthy London Partnership. Mental health crisis care for Londoners: London's section 136 pathway and Health Based Place of Safety specification [Online]. 2017. Available at: https://www.healthylondon.org/wp-content/uploads/2017/10/Londons-section-136-pathway-and-HBPoS-specification-updated-Dec-2017.pdf
15. Clements C, Turnbull P, Hawton K, Geulayov G, Waters K, Ness J, Townsend E, Khundakar K, Kapur N. Rates of self-harm presenting to general hospitals: a comparison of data from the multicentre study of self-harm in England and hospital episode statistics. BMJ Open. 2016;6(2):e009749.
16. Hawton K, Bergen H, Casey D, Simkin S, Palmer B, Cooper J, Kapur N, Horrocks J, House A, Lilley R, Noble R, Owens D. Self-harm in England: a tale of three cities. Soc Psychiatry Psychiatr Epidemiol. 2007;42(7):513–21.
17. Royal College of Emergency Medicine. Frequent attenders in the emergency department [Online]. 2017. Available at: https://www.rcem.ac.uk/docs/RCEM%20Guidance/Guideline%20-%20Frequent%20Attenders%20in%20the%20ED%20(Aug%202017).pdf
18. Greenfield G, Blair M, Aylin PP, Saxena S, Majeed A, Hoffman M, Bottle A. Frequent attendances at emergency departments in England. Emerg Med J. 2020;37(10):597–9.
19. Health and Social Care Act 2008 (Regulated Activities) Regulations. 2014. Available at: https://www.legislation.gov.uk/ukdsi/2014/9780111117613/contents

Approved Mental Health Professional

Mary Brazier

1   Introduction

This chapter provides the reader with an understanding of how the role of the Approved Mental Health Professional (AMHP) interfaces with other emergency clinicians. Three anonymised case examples illustrate how the different agencies and roles work together and the importance of a full understanding of roles and responsibilities at all levels in delivering care to people experiencing acute mental illness.

2   AMHP Role and Responsibilities

The Approved Mental Health Professional or 'AMHP' is a role created in the 2007 amendments to the Mental Health Act 1983 [1]; previous to these amendments, the role was that of the Approved Social Worker, and it has been referred to as '…critical to the operation of the Mental Health Act' [2]. AMHPs act on behalf of local authorities to carry out a variety of functions under the MHA. One key responsibility is to make applications for the detention of individuals in hospital, ensuring both the MHA and its Code of Practice is followed. It is the AMHP's duty, when two medical recommendations have been made, to decide whether or not to make the application for the detention of the person who has been assessed under the MHA, this process is often colloquially also known as 'sectioning'. This includes considering the relevant legal frameworks: the Mental Capacity Act [3], including Deprivation of Liberty Safeguards, whether there are any least restrictive alternatives to admission, ensuring that the patient is involved and identifying and involving their Nearest Relative [2].

M. Brazier (✉)
Director of Social Work, East London NHS Foundation Trust, London, UK
e-mail: Mary.Brazier@nhs.net

T. Scott (ed.), *Mental Health: Intervention Skills for the Emergency Services*,
https://doi.org/10.1007/978-3-031-20347-3_7

The AMHP provides an independent decision about whether or not there are alternatives to detention under the Act, seeking the least restrictive alternative and bringing a social perspective to bear on their decision [4]. Therefore, the role of the AMHP is a complex one, encompassing a range of responsibilities with regard to the coordination and undertaking of assessments under the MHA. These duties are set out in s13 of the MHA. Arguably, the most important element of the role of the AMHP concerns making the application for the detention of a patient following the MHA Assessment. Making the decision to detain someone to hospital where they may be treated against their will could be considered difficult and challenging. Also, significant logistical challenges and practical and emotional tensions held by the AMHP interplay, including having the detained person in their custody for the period between the legal detention papers being completed and the person being formally 'accepted' by the hospital, on occasion this period of time can be a number of hours.

Whilst the 2007 amendments opened the role to other registered professions, namely, registered mental health nurses, occupational therapists and psychologists, the role remains largely undertaken by social workers. A 2020 survey of local authorities found that 95% of all AMHPs were social workers [5]. The circumstances and contexts of MHA assessments are many and varied, as they can take place in people's own homes, in acute hospitals, on inpatient wards and in emergency departments. They can also take place in police custody where people have been arrested for an offence before a mental health need becomes apparent, as well as in 'health-based places of safety' for those detained under s135 or s136 of the MHA and brought to those locations for assessment. There are no upper or lower age limits for MHA assessments; indeed, the author has been involved with assessments for older people in their late 90s as well as pre-teen children.

3 Interagency Cooperation

The complexity of assessments under the MHA, as well as the range of circumstances in which they can take place, means that joint working is inevitable; interagency cooperation and understanding are therefore key to making this joint working effective in delivering the most appropriate care for the individuals involved. Without a shared sense of purpose and understanding of how different professionals and agencies exercise different powers, limitations, roles and responsibilities, there is a risk that these most challenging of interventions become mired in misunderstanding and frustration.

How to achieve interagency cooperation in a way that ensures effective functioning at the point-of-care delivery is a vital question to be answered in each local health and social care system. The Mental Health Act Code of Practice [6] states that:

> The objective of local partnership arrangements is to ensure that people experiencing mental health crisis receive the right medical care from the most appropriate health agencies as

soon as possible. The Police will often, due to the nature of their role, be the first point of contact for individuals in crisis, but it is crucial that people experiencing mental health crisis access appropriate health services at the earliest opportunity.

Producing, agreeing and formally signing such interagency agreements on behalf of each organisation are one thing, but the agreements are, first and foremost, working documents that need to make sense to all who refer to them. It is therefore important to ensure that the local joint agreement can be used easily in practice and that it does not sit in the electronic version of a dusty folder; it should include clear pathways and responsibilities, clear processes for escalation and identification of key decision-makers. If a patient is in the emergency department when they need to be conveyed to a specialist mental health facility, it is important to assign responsibility for ensuring that barriers to the timely transfer are removed and that the needs of the patient are met whilst those arrangements are being made, and for escalation routes in case of ongoing barriers. It is imperative that the Mental Health Trust provides appropriate support enabled by safe mental health nurse staffing levels. It is also important to explore whether the patient can be transferred to a health-based place of safety, who explores these options and who needs to be involved to make decisions and authorise actions. Not all of the elements of the joint working protocols will be relevant to all agencies, all professionals and all clinicians, but they should all know of its existence and location in order to refer to it on the occasions when it is needed. The occasions which require problem-solving processes to be most effective are by their very nature the most complex, with associated expressions of escalated emotions often focused on perceived inaction or delay on the part of others.

Another way to facilitate and encourage good interagency joint working, understanding, and cooperation is multiagency training. The opportunity to bring frontline and patient-facing staff from different agencies together to work through various scenarios is an important one; it enables the joint working protocol to be tested in scenario-based teaching and learning across agencies, and by doing so, it facilitates understanding between individuals at various levels of seniority within organisations. MHA assessments, perceptions of delay or inappropriate responses from different organisations often happen during periods of high stress when individuals express heightened emotion. The opportunity to build good working relationships on a less formal basis and talk through scenarios from different perspectives enables understanding which, it is hoped, is useful 'on the ground'; furthermore, it helps to avoid difficult conversations at the worst possible times. It is understandable that in times of high expressed emotion, in cases of particular complexity, if there is not a shared understanding of roles and responsibilities, this may be expressed in terms of more difficult conversations, uncertainty about roles and what to do next expressed as grumpiness or unhelpfulness, perceived barriers to moving forward rather than an understanding of circumstances outside the control of the individual. As practitioners we are largely, for understandable reasons, preoccupied with our own function and responsibilities, what **we** have to achieve, sometimes 'spinning too many plates' with regard a number of different factors which all need to be in place for a successful resolution for the person experiencing mental health crisis. As AMHPs and the professional responsible for coordinating the assessment, we are often concerned firstly with the logistics and are likely to have a number of concerns in mind on arrival at the agreed location:

- Will everyone turn up at the right time in the right place?
- Will the person be in?
- I haven't heard about the bed yet; I hope there is one.
- I hope there isn't a delay in the ambulance attending.

If the Mental Health Act Assessment has taken place in the person's own home, this may well have gone ahead prior to the AMHP knowing where the person would be admitted, if indeed the outcome of the assessment is that an admission is the most appropriate 'least restrictive' alternative. The AMHP will be undertaking their own assessment of the needs of the person, liaising with the relevant family and friends, identifying the nearest relative (s26 MHA), and, often, will be asking very personal and potentially intrusive questions of those present, who are themselves likely to be distressed both due to the circumstances themselves and the processes involved.

It is important that the AMHPs have an understanding of the thoughts and priorities of the other professionals as it can often feel that all the responsibility is being held by this one person, whereas it is likely that the different people attending are also experiencing the same thoughts. Indeed, it is possible that paramedics and police who may be on site for lengthy periods could be prevented from responding to other priority calls. If the assessment is taking place in an ED, it is critical that the AMHP and the s12 (MHA) Approved Doctors understand the challenges faced by the clinicians in the department, as they balance the needs of very physically and mentally unwell people, together with organising the care of someone who in their view possibly shouldn't be there. When AMHPs experience these situations, there is a risk that there are different perspectives on how to resolve the problem, extending even to different views on what the actual 'problem' might be. So, it is of utmost importance that the person with mental health needs does not become perceived to be 'the problem', even when planning for their treatment or care. Practising hypothetical scenarios within a safe teaching environment is therefore incredibly useful, if not essential.

The other vital element to good joint working practice is a regular interagency forum to discuss, deconstruct, and resolve issues. In the Thames Valley area of England this is known as 'Partnerships in Practice', with attendees from the various statutory and nonstatutory agencies. The relationships formed by the agency representatives are useful in themselves in terms of mutual support in finding solutions to complex situations. On the ground concerns about, for example, whose job it is and who takes responsibility for particular actions are important aspects which need clarification. Fundamentally, such fora can facilitate positive, proactive networks of practitioners and agencies working together to ensure whole system effectiveness.

Whenever multiple agencies come together at the point-of-care delivery, there is the potential for miscommunication, misunderstanding and frustration. To put some of these issues into practice, it is helpful to think through them using a case study approach which considers different scenarios and roles.

3.1   Case Study: Julia

Julia, a 26-year-old woman, attended the emergency department of the local acute hospital having made cuts to her arms whilst significantly intoxicated. Whilst awaiting further medical assessment, Julia left the department. As a result of significant concerns about her risk to herself, ED clinicians contacted the local police to report their concerns. Julia was found by police in the grounds of the hospital, whereby officers assessed that the criteria for use of s136 (1) MHA were met[1] and she was detained by them; following local arrangements, an ambulance was called, and Julia was then taken to a health-based place of safety at the local mental health unit. Once in the health-based place of safety, the nursing staff made a referral to the Approved Mental Health Professional Service for a MHA Assessment by an AMHP and two s12 Approved Doctors, the outcome of which was that Julia was no longer intoxicated, was engaging with the assessing team and was keen to accept support from community services to address her difficulties with alcohol dependency. Julia was clear with the AMHP and doctors that she had not experienced suicidal thoughts and had no plans to end her life but became very distressed the night before and for a number of years had responded to distress by making cuts to her arms, which she described as helping 'release the pressure'. Appointments were therefore made with the local alcohol service and the community mental health team, and Julia returned home in a taxi organised by the AMHP. As a result of the cuts to her arm not receiving attention previously, Julia also needed to see her general practitioner for further care.

In the above case study, Julia's journey may be reflected upon. She had contact with the ED, police service, ambulance service, health-based place of safety staff, the AMHP and s12 doctors, all within a short period of time, and each asked her what had happened because they have different functions under the MHA and clinically. It is useful to reflect on how different professionals may interact with Julia given her presenting needs resulted from self-inflicted physical harm and her subsequent departure from the department before she was assessed and treated. Julia's presentation is not unusual, often seen in people given a diagnosis of 'emotionally unstable personality disorder'. How to appropriately support people who seek help in this way can present a challenge to services as they have more recently been categorised as 'high-intensity users' reflecting the statistic that as much as 70% of this demand is caused by a small number of 'high-intensity users' who struggle with complex trauma and behavioural disorders [7]. Service responses which have attempted to address this disproportionate contact with services are often, however, subject to challenge and criticism, particularly those which sought to embed police officers within mental health services. Criticism of this model of practice arose

---

[1] S136 (1) If a person appears to a constable to be suffering from mental disorder and to be in immediate need of care or control, the constable may, if he thinks necessary to do so in the interests of that person or for the protection of other persons :

(a) Remove the person to a place of safety within the meaning of S135.
(b) If the person is already at a place of safety within the meaning of that section, keep the person at that place or remove the person to another place of safety.

regarding their lack of evidence base and apparent focus on reducing what is perceived as 'inappropriate'. A 2005 study explored the reasons why almost half of people presenting to general hospitals after an incident of self-harm did not stay to enable a full psychosocial assessment to be undertaken [8]. A number of factors were identified; however, males were at increased risk of suicide compared with females; those who had taken illegal drugs or/and alcohol and those attending 'out of hours' were more likely to self-discharge.

Agreeing the most appropriate way to support people who present in mental health crisis to EDs is incredibly complex and controversial. The role of the police in circumstances where the person presents with ambivalence, seeking help and then leaving the department prior to care being given, is also often misunderstood. Officers can be asked to assist with restraint in order for treatment to be given and to remain in case the person becomes agitated or tries to leave. The desire to seek an authoritative presence may be understandable, but officers have no legal powers in these circumstances other than the use of s136 MHA to remove the person to a health-based place of safety. Unanswered questions remain regarding how best to keep a person safe, and whose responsibility it is, until they are in the most appropriate place for them. This provides another example where interagency relationships and agreements are vital. In cases such as these, it is important that no assumptions are made and that until a formal transfer of responsibility has been agreed and documented, then that transfer of responsibility has not taken place. A tragic example highlighting the importance of effective transfer of care and understanding of local joint working protocols is illustrated in the case of a man who died by suicide after leaving an acute hospital ED in circumstances where responsibility for his care had not been agreed between staff from different agencies.[2]

Given all the different points of contact for Julia in this case study, it is important to consider how the information obtained during each of those contacts is passed on to the next point of contact. In this example, Julia was seen by staff from the emergency department, police officers, ambulance crew and staff at the health-based place of safety prior to seeing the AMHP and the s12 doctors. Often, by the time the MHA Assessment takes place, a lot of that information may not be available, leaving the person to tell their story again. Each of those professionals will have obtained information from Julia or observed different incidents; they may have kept a written note of their contact in their own records, but it is important to consider how that information may be available to the AMHP and the s12 doctors, who are undertaking their assessment in a new location for the person, who may no longer appear to be distressed. It is in the interests of the person for the AMHP and s12 doctors to have at least an overview of what happened at the point of the decision to use s136, often very limited information is passed on via the local agency documentation and the AMHP rarely has an opportunity to speak directly with the detaining police officer.

---

[2] https://www.judiciary.uk/wp-content/uploads/2014/08/Church-2014-0331.pdf

3.2   Case Study: David

The local AMHP service received a referral from a Community Mental Health Team (CMHT) regarding David, a patient of the team. The referral outlined that David had a diagnosis of schizophrenia, and his care plan included a fortnightly injection of a long-acting antipsychotic medication. David did not attend his most recent two clinic appointments, and family members reported that he had begun to express paranoid thoughts that others were seeking to harm him, he was refusing most food and drink and would not allow others into his home. The CMHT had been unable to gain access despite a number of visits to David's home. The referral requested MHA Assessment to consider admission to hospital for his treatment regime to be restarted. The AMHPs considered the referral taking into account the potential risks to the patient of not ingesting adequate nutrition for over a week and refusing contact with professionals and family members. Subsequently, the AMHPs applied to the magistrates for a warrant s135(1) MHA, which on receipt of supporting evidence was granted. To execute the warrant, the AMHP coordinated the attendance of the police, ambulance and a s12 MHA approved doctor. On arrival at the address and after the AMHP had liaised with the family and explained about the plan to use the warrant they enabled access by opening the door. On entering the property, David had locked himself in his bathroom and refused to come out to speak with the AMHP and the s12 doctor, who spent time talking to him through the bathroom door. Eventually, they persuaded David to open the door, at which time the police officer encouraged him to go with the ambulance personnel who subsequently transported him to the designated health-based place of safety located at the local mental health inpatient unit, for a further assessment to be undertaken.

A number of important factors should be considered in the above case study. The execution of warrants under the MHA is a particularly complex process indeed, in many ways it is deemed the most complex piece of work undertaken under the MHA. It requires significant coordination between agencies as, in order for a warrant to be executed, an AMHP, a s12 approved doctor, a police officer and an ambulance need to be in the same place at the same time. Each of those services has competing operational demands and priorities.

In order for the warrant to be obtained, the AMHP must satisfy a magistrate that the criteria as set out in s135(1) are met. The AMHP will have written a report for the court outlining why the person meets the criteria:

…that there is reasonable cause to suspect that a person believed to be suffering from mental disorder -

a) Has been, or is being, ill-treated, neglected or kept otherwise than under proper control, in any place within the jurisdiction of the justice, or

b) Being unable to care for himself, is living alone in any such place, the justice may issue a warrant…

The information presented to the court will therefore have included why the person is considered to need an assessment under the MHA and what other options have been attempted prior to the use of a warrant. The court needs to be satisfied that the criteria are met and will have read the written evidence presented by the AMHP as well as been able to question the AMHP directly under oath about their evidence.

On obtaining the warrant from the magistrate's court, the AMHP will then have coordinated the attendance of the various agencies in this case, police officer, s12 doctor and ambulance practitioner often together with family members or other key holders to facilitate access to the property. This, in itself, is one of the most time-consuming elements of executing a s135(1) warrant. Therefore, on arriving at the property, for other professionals, this is their first knowledge of the person involved, but for the AMHP(s), this case has already been afforded significant investment of time and negotiation, meeting at the property being the culmination of that work. At this point as a result, the AMHP will hold valuable information. Taking time at this stage to talk through the reasons for being present and how the execution of the warrant might progress including who will take the lead with communication is important. In practical terms, agreeing to meet away from the property to ensure all involved are briefed fully can be useful to avoid causing distress to the occupant. Each professional present has a distinct role in the execution of the warrant and the mental health assessment of the individual concerned. It is very important that the distinction between the different roles is understood and mutually respected.

The execution of a warrant can also be an emotionally as well as practically complex intervention. The power to force entry into the home of someone experiencing significant mental ill-health is one which, whilst never used lightly, has a significant impact on the person themselves; it feels an incredibly intrusive and on occasions violent intervention if force has to be used. If the person is already frightened and possibly paranoid, the forced entry of professionals can further fuel those fears. Practical challenges need to be considered, not least of which is protecting the privacy and dignity of the person who may be in significant distress. The arrival of a number of vehicles and uniformed professionals some of which will be clearly identifiable frequently generates the interest of neighbours who may approach the people in attendance to ask what is happening. Indeed, neighbours may be aware of aspects of the person's history and may wish to communicate this.

It is desirable that people experiencing significant mental health needs are able to engage with the voluntary assessment and treatment process where possible. However, in those cases where the person is not able to do so for whichever reason and is unwilling, the warrant provides legislative powers to remove the person from their property and states when and how this may happen. If the mentally unwell person is refusing or is reluctant to do so, an incredibly difficult decision arises. Often the person may be 'busying themselves' appearing to be making preparation but in effect delaying the inevitable time when they will need to leave their home. For the AMHP and other professionals, knowing when to support the individual through the process of preparing to leave their home, by helping them to gather specific items that are important to them and that they may wish to take with them, and leave feeling confident that their home will be safe in their absence and when to say 'we're going now' is one that requires skill, diplomacy and confidence, particularly when the latter stage may require professionals to put 'hands on'. When to transition from encouragement and support to a more physical intervention is a difficult decision to make and needs to be done following discussion between all present and an agreement as to how the intervention can be completed whilst maximising the privacy and dignity of the person.

3.3   Case Study: Brenda

A 92-year-old woman, Brenda, recently returned to her own home following a 3-week stay in a nursing home where she had been receiving rehabilitation following an inpatient admission in the local acute hospital following a chest infection. Brenda had been supplied with domiciliary support, to meet her identified care and support needs; she was visited four times each day by two carers to assist her to maintain her personal hygiene and nutrition and prompt her to take her medication. She was referred to the CMHT for older people by her GP who had undertaken a home visit, to find Brenda in a poor physical state, apparently incontinent of urine and faeces, and the GP was concerned for her mental state due to how confused, distressed and agitated Brenda was. The care agency also expressed concern due to her refusal to allow the domiciliary carers to support her and as described by them to be '…throwing items at the carers and insisting they leave her home'. Following an initial visit to Brenda at home, the community psychiatric nurse (CPN) noted that the Brenda was presenting in the way described by the GP and was also concerned about the risk of fire as Brenda tended to smoke cigarettes in bed, as had been her practice for many years.

The CMHT discussed Brenda's case with the AMHPs, to explore whether MHA Assessment was appropriate in these circumstances. The AMHPs considered the referral then suggested that an assessment under the Mental Capacity Act [3] could be used and then outlined the processes for the CMHT to follow should Brenda lack the capacity to consent to going to hospital and having treatment. In this instance a decision to go ahead could be made in her best interests. However, the paramedics were reluctant to follow this course of action given the degree of objection expressed by Brenda. In the meantime, a number of different agencies became involved with attempting to support Brenda: her general practitioner, adult social care, the care agency and the CMHT. All the agencies reported increasing concern about a deterioration in Brenda's physical health that her skin was looking increasingly red and appeared to be irritating her as she constantly scratched, she was eating very little and did not take prescribed medication even though she reported significant pain. It was believed that her confusion was likely to be caused by delirium, but that further assessment in a medical ward was required to confirm this and treat any identified cause.

The CMHT called the ambulance service to support Brenda's admission to the acute hospital. On arrival, paramedics had significant difficulty persuading her to agree to go with them, given her ongoing degree of confusion. A request for police assistance to support her physical removal was considered; however, they were unable to attend. After some hours, paramedics encouraged her onto a stretcher and transferred her into the ambulance. On arrival into the ED, Brenda's level of agitation continued, and then she was admitted onto a ward for treatment of cellulitis. Her diagnosis was confirmed as 'delirium secondary to infection'. As she did not have the capacity to consent, Brenda's inpatient admission was authorised under the Deprivation of Liberty Safeguards, and her treatment was given under the MCA.

On reflection, the main challenge in planning the way forward with Brenda's presentation was determining the most applicable legal framework. When someone presents with delirium, as was the assumption in this case with a sudden onset of confusion and agitation in the context of a likely infection, there is the option of using the MCA to convey the person to hospital and treat them within an acute hospital. However, professionals are sometimes reluctant to commit to such a decision in these circumstances, being less confident regarding the legal powers afforded by the MCA, particularly when there is a significant and or physical objection. In this case there was an attempt to involve police, based on the assumption that police have powers beyond other disciplines. Whilst in this case police were unable to attend, it is useful to recognise that the police service is only able to act where they have an explicit power to do so. In the above example, police had no more powers than any other professional; given the plan to use the MCA, the professionals already in attendance had the powers they needed.

Application of the MCA in this way is often a secondary consideration, when the most usual course of action where someone's main presentation of concern as regards their behaviour is to use the MHA; it can become the default in these circumstances. The AMHP role in this case was to provide advice and guidance as regards the MCA and the powers within. This case study also illustrates how many different professionals with different roles and responsibilities can intervene with one person, sometimes in the same place, as in the example of the CPN from the CMHT, attending the home with the care agency following a GP referral, the consultation with the AMHPs, the attendance of the paramedics and the attempt to involve police.

Again, this is an example of where shared understanding was really important in ensuring the person ultimately received the right intervention in the right place, at the right time. What is less visible in the case study is the role of the emergency department in Brenda's journey from her home onto a medical ward. It is important to consider what interventions the emergency department practitioners should consider to minimise distress and confusion for Brenda. The decision to use the MCA in her own home should be conveyed accurately and appropriately to the department; and identification of the person whose role it would be to ensure that this takes place should be confirmed. Further, emergency clinicians should know what the admission plan might be, not only from the perspective of clinical assessment, diagnosis and intervention but also regarding the legal frameworks which enable and allow intervention when someone lacks the capacity to consent.

4 Conclusion

The intent with this chapter has been to demonstrate how the circumstances of people presenting with mental health needs have the potential to be complex, not just in terms of clinical presentation but also in terms of inter-professional and interagency relationships and communication. In order to deliver effective interventions, the understanding of each other's roles and responsibilities and the skills to communicate effectively at all times are key.

Learning Points
- Explain your role when you attend a Mental Health Act Assessment.
- Identify the lead clinician responsible for Mental Health Liaison in your speciality.
- Explain how you would you escalate points of concern or clarification (i) in your organisation and (ii) to the wider system.

References

1. GOV.UK. 2007 amendments to the Mental Health Act. 1983. https://www.legislation.gov.uk/ukpga/2007/12/contents
2. Care Quality Commission. Mental health act: approved mental health professional services. Mar 2018. https://www.cqc.org.uk/sites/default/files/20180326_mha_amhpbriefing.pdf
3. Mental Capacity Act. Crown copyright. London. 2005. https://www.legislation.gov.uk/ukpga/2005/9/contents. Accessed 20 Jan 2022.
4. Department of Health. Code of practice: mental health act 1983. London: Department of Health; 2008. p. 4.51.
5. DHSC, Skills for Care, and Workforce Intelligence. The Approved Mental Health Professional in the adult social care sector. Feb 2021. https://www.skillsforcare.org.uk/adult-social-care-workforce-data/Workforce-intelligence/documents/AMHPs-Briefing.pdf
6. MHA Code of Practice. 16:30. 2015. https://assets.publishing.service.gov.uk/government/uploads/system/uploads/attachment_data/file/435512/MHA_Code_of_Practice.PDF#:~:text=Mental%20Health%20Act%201983%3A%20Code%20of%20Practice%20.,restrictive%20interventions%2C%20seclusion%2C%20use%20of%20police%20powers%20to
7. Turner S. The High Intensity Network (HIN) approach and SIM model for mental health care and 'high intensity users'–what are your views? 2021. https://highintensitynetwork.org/#:~:text=High%20Intensity%20Network%20Across%20the%20UK%2C%20emergency%20and,who%20struggle%20with%20complex%20trauma%20and%20behavioural%20disorders%3F. Accessed 31 Mar 2022.
8. Bennewith O, Peters TJ, Hawton K, House A, Gunnell D. Factors associated with the non-assessment of self-harm patients attending an accident and emergency department: results of a national study. J Affect Disord. 2005;89(1–3):91–7.

Children and Young Peoples' Services

Gemma Trainor and Shelley O'Connor

1 Introduction

Mental health problems are often central issues affecting young people in today's society. Epidemiological data indicate that 50% of all major psychiatric conditions excluding dementia are diagnosable by the age of 14 [1], yet, despite significant improvements in legislation and policy, services for young people remain disjointed, underfunded and varied across the four nations of the United Kingdom. Over recent years there have been major advances in how mental health of children and young people (CYP) including emergency services is addressed and managed in the United Kingdom. Among these ambitions is the *Future in Mind* report [2] which recommended how to improve the current state of affairs across CYP in England. Concurrently, there has been significant investment in early intervention, waiting time initiatives and locating Child and Adolescent Mental Health Services (CAMHS) in schools over a 5-year period. The lack of coordination between services is included in these innovative transformational plans with the aim of reducing the burden on acute services and promotes access to the right service at the right time.

In Wales, *Together for Children and Young People* (T4CYP) was launched in 2015 prioritising CYP's emotional and mental health [3]. With government cross-cabinet commitment, this multiagency service improvement programme considers ways to reshape, remodel and refocus emotional and mental health services provided for CYP in Wales. The original 4-year programme was extended to 2021 and of the work streams of T4CYP involves reviewing the roles of community and specialist CAMH services.

G. Trainor (✉) · S. O'Connor
Liverpool John Moores University, Liverpool, UK
e-mail: g.trainor@ljmu.ac.uk; s.b.oconnor@ljmu.ac.uk

T. Scott (ed.), *Mental Health: Intervention Skills for the Emergency Services*, https://doi.org/10.1007/978-3-031-20347-3_8

The Scottish Government and the Convention of Scottish Local Authorities (COSLA) identified the need to focus on the mental well-being of CYP in the *Getting It Right for Every Child (GIRFEC)* document [4] which was designed to also ensure CYP receive the right help at the right time from the right people. The Scottish Government Mental Health Strategy 2017–2027 [5] also included reforms on early intervention, prevention and addressing regional variations.

The Northern Ireland Commissioner for Children and Young people (NICCY) launched *Still Waiting* [6] in 2018, a rights-based review of the adequacy of mental health services and support for CYP. Recommendations called for a regional model with transformation to pathways and referral processes included but not exhaustive: mandatory mental health training for all professionals, designated healthcare professionals, a combination of streamlined emergency care and community services, monitoring waiting times and an integrated mental health service model for CYP inclusive of those with a learning disability. Despite the anticipation of the report and its action plan, changes to the current system have been slow due to funding uncertainty (Northern Ireland Commissioner for Children and Young People [7].

New data has emerged as to the prevalence of mental health disorders in young people being more than previously thought in that 12.8% (1 in 8) of those young people aged between 5 and 19 had at least one mental disorder, an increase on the previous estimate of 1 in 10 [8]. This survey of 9117 children in England with a diagnosable mental health disorder showed that 1 in 12 had an emotional disorder (anxiety, depression) with higher rates among girls (10.2%) compared to boys (6.2%). It is the first time pre-school children have been included, and a stark 1 in 18 (5.5%) was identified with at least one disorder such as behavioural disorder or autistic spectrum disorder (ASD). Among ages 5 to 10, disorders were more common among boys (12.2%) than girls (6.6%).

Furthermore, between 2004 and 2017, there was an alarming increase in self-harm rates particularly among females. Some groups of young people are more vulnerable than others such as looked after children who have more complex needs. Therefore, early recognition and prompt referrals can help reduce the default to crisis and urgent care presentations. However, identifying and responding appropriately to the mental health needs of CYP can prove challenging to emergency service practitioners who may not feel fully equipped to handle these encounters. Child and Adolescent Mental Health Services (CAMHS) is provided through a network of services organised in four tiers, and the roles of the different tiers in England are shown below. Similar arrangements exist in Wales, Scotland and Northern Ireland.

2   Tier 1

Services provided by practitioners in universal services (such as early years services, primary care, health visitors, school nurses, teachers and youth workers) who are non-specialists who can:

- Offer general advice in certain cases
- Administer treatment for less severe problems
- Promote mental health
- Aid early identification of problems
- Refer to specialist services

3   Tier 2

A service provided by specialist individuals such as youth offending teams, primary mental health workers and school and youth counselling (including social care and education) who offer:

- Training and consultation for other professionals
- Consultation for families and carers
- Outreach to families and children requiring more help, who are unwilling to use specialist services
- Assessment, which may trigger further treatment

4   Tier 3

A specialist multidisciplinary service for more severe, complex or persistent disorders, offering:

- Assessment and treatment
- Assessment for referrals to tier 4
- Contributions to consultation and training at tiers 1 and 2
- Participation in research and development projects

5   Tier 4

These are specialist tertiary services comprising:

• Day units
• Highly specialist inpatient and outpatient services

Most young people do not receive specialist services and can be managed in low-level mental health services (i.e. CAMHS tier 1 and 2 services), such as schools, third sector and local authority children's services. For that reason, it is imperative that all healthcare and statutory staff should have a sound understanding of how to assess and address the emotional well-being of CYP. At the very least, all professionals responding to a crisis should be able to recognise if a child is suffering with a mental health problem and liaise with the appropriate services. Mental health promotion should be the underpinning principle as well as the promotion of psychological and emotional well-being of children and their families/carers.

Additionally, staff should be mindful of the potential factors that can put a child at risk [9, 10]. There are a myriad of risk factors and, although interrelated, these can be loosely classified into individual, family and social. The individual factors range from psychiatric illness, major depressive disorder, suicidal behaviour and psychosis to general feelings of hopelessness, disappointment or anger, a tendency to be impulsive, a lack of insight into their limitations, impaired social skills and an inability to solve problems. Substance abuse is a particular risk factor as is experience of domestic violence or abuse (physical, emotional and sexual). Family factors include relationship difficulties or disordered attachment, separation, divorce or bereavement and forms of abuse. Social factors comprise criminality or unemployment, poor relationships with peer group and bullying which can lead to isolation or exclusion.

This chapter is aimed at emergency services practitioners who work with young people, to help them identify the skills and knowledge they need to respond appropriately. This may also assist in developing local guidelines to operate alongside national recommendations (e.g. National Institute for Health and Care Excellence (NICE) guidance) for the safe and effective care of these vulnerable CYP.

6   Mental Health Crisis

There is often a cross over between social and mental health care which is rarely due to a mental health crisis alone. Such episodes tend to occur when the level of distress cannot be managed within the young person's current situation or the community in which they live. The precise circumstances could be gleaned from the opinion of the young person, the parents/carers or the view of others involved in their care. It could be that the young person or others consider their condition may be worsening or that they can no longer cope safely and may be at imminent risk of harm to themselves or others, so help is sought. The crisis service comprises any service that is available at short notice to help the young person by providing support to resolve the crisis. CAMHS crisis and intensive service models have also undergone significant change with a move away from inpatient CAMH services to alternative provision such as intensive outpatient and outreach services.

There is a plethora of evidence of the benefits of liaison psychiatric services, and the composition of the team is described in guides such as *NHS England achieve better access to 24/7 urgent and emergency care* [11]. Currently it is advised that all acute trusts provide liaison psychiatric services over a 24-hour period, although CAMHS have some catching up to do if they are to address deficiencies as currently young people are being inappropriately assessed by adult psychiatric services. Services differ across the four countries of the United Kingdom, and for some young people, they might not acquire access to screening by CAMHS, and for others there may be an avoidable delay.

Mental health disorders among children and adolescents are increasing, attributing to 16% of the global burden of disease and injury [12] which has recently been compounded by the COVID-19 pandemic. By ignoring a rise in cases now, mental health conditions will likely exacerbate and continue through to adulthood, affecting physical and mental health and quality of life. To reduce the level of burden on healthcare professionals and healthcare services and provide a linear and timely support structure for children and adolescents and their families, a multidisciplinary, co-ordinated and integrated care pathway is crucial. Frontline emergency services ought to provide an agile and pragmatic response, yet this support is often fraught with issues in times of crisis compounded by a lack of resources.

In a 2018 audit of child and adolescent crisis admissions from EDs to CAMHS beds in the South London and Maudsley NHS Foundation Trust area, 71 CYP of which 40 were admitted informally and 31 under the Mental Health Act (1983 amended in 2007), 62% presented with self-harm, suicide or emotional dysregulation. This built on the previous year when the figure was 38 patients via crisis admission. Duration of waiting times between ED attendance to CAMHS bed increased, figures were reported at 2 days (pre-2017) and an average of 4 days (post-2017) [13]. Bed occupancy and a shrinking workforce were reported as particularly challenging to mental health services. Without sufficient levels of frontline staff and a lack of resources, the burden falls on EDs to cope with crisis attendances and admissions.

The Mental Health Liaison Psychiatry team residing within EDs currently support CYP because CAMHS specialist services do not operate within EDs. There is however a commitment following the Mental Health Crisis Care Concordat to provide 24-hour liaison psychiatry services by 2023/2024 in England and Wales, yet this will only feature in 70% of acute hospitals despite attendance rates rising. Mental health provision for CYP remains under-resourced, and problems around timely assessments and inability to access CAMHS beds remain. According to the Royal College of Emergency Medicine (RCEM), liaison psychiatry teams should undergo training by CAMHS teams to strengthen risk assessment of a CYP and to decide if he/she should stay in hospital or be discharged home followed by a full assessment from a CAMHS team [14], yet there is little evidence that this training occurs.

7   Right Care at the Right Time

The introduction of the new care models programme, a key component of the *NHS Five Year Forward View for Mental Health*, was introduced in England in 2016, featuring delegates of whole pathway management to local healthcare economies, to maximise impact for patients using services. Northumberland Accountable Care Organisation aimed to integrate primary and acute care systems by promoting effective working and a shared vision. The opening of the Northumbria Specialist Emergency Care Hospital in June 2015 transformed urgent and emergency care, closely followed up by locality based multidisciplinary teams (MDT) supporting patients in their homes and reducing the number of crisis and hospital admissions. The Leicester, Leicestershire and Rutland System Resilience group aim was to improve the coordination of urgent and emergency care services, offering a 24/7 service to improve information sharing and signposting between services. The *Mental Health Alliance for Excellence, Resilience, Innovation and Training (MERIT)* providing specialist mental health services in the West Midlands was set up to improve efficiency, with a focus on crisis care and risk reduction, recovery and rehabilitation. The overarching aim was that service users should benefit from a coordinated emergency response, timely decision-making and shared care plans among professionals which was advocated to reduce distress and repetition for service users [15].

The *NHS Long-Term Plan* [16] acknowledges a gap in mental health services for CYP and the pressure on emergency services, despite the efforts of frontline workers. The number of CYP accessing community mental health services has risen from 325,000 in 2017/2018 to almost 380,000 in 2018/2019 [17] with almost 27,000 emergency admissions due to self-harm in 10 to 19-year-olds in 2017/2018 [18]. Overstretched crisis services mean that CYP do not receive the help they need and this escalation has seen a sharp increase in emergency admissions, far from a therapeutic environment.

A busy emergency department is unlikely to be conducive to providing clinicians with a suitable physical environment where a healthy therapeutic exchange may take place. There should be adequate space or a room away from public areas and the waiting room so that the young person and their families/carers can feel accepted, safe, secure and understood, so that they can experience unconditional positive regard to be able to verbalise and consider their thoughts more fully about the episode. Therefore, as the young person is the client and, wherever possible, they should be seen first, after which, practitioners can interview parents/carers to corroborate the risk assessment and to draw up a safety plan. The safety plan will often require the adults to be part of the solution for ensuring the young person's safety. In a survey conducted by YoungMinds of 1531 parents with children who had experienced a mental health crisis found that 86% felt access prior to the crisis would have been helpful, and 65% agreed that access to a crisis telephone hotline would have supported them also [19].

8   Management of Mental Health Crises

Emergency services personnel are not necessarily equipped to support and manage CYP in a mental health crisis, yet do so with passion and resolve. Despite the negative coverage they receive, they play a vital role in supporting CYP:

> Today is my 1 year since my last and most serious suicide attempt. I am thankful to the stranger, the police, and paramedics that saved my life that night. Because of you I have a future. (Tweet on Twitter, 2021)

Emergency services personnel are frontline workers involved in emergency management who encompass those working in the healthcare sector: paramedics, ED doctors/nurses, police and fire service, responding to situations that require immediate response, to those in imminent danger. Mental health crisis can unfold as scenes of self-harm, suicidal intent, unusual mental state or a psychiatric emergency [20]. It is a common occurrence among CYP to experience crisis that can often lead to adult mental health problems, especially if not dealt with correctly. More often, it is the first time a CYP has presented themselves to mental health services, so the help they receive can have a long-lasting impression on them.

The Policing and Mental Health document *Picking Up the Pieces* suggests that despite the considerate, supportive and compassionate approach of the general police force, there is a glitch in the system with a lack of support in primary care and early intervention to prevent the flux of mental health crises.

As Sir Thomas Winsor, Her Majesty's Chief Inspector of Constabulary said in his 2017 *State of Policing* report:

> There will always be situations where someone in crisis needs a rapid response from the emergency services. But too often, our public services are failing to work together to prevent the crisis in the first place … Blue lights should not have to flash for someone to get the help they need in time [21].

9   Professional Attitudes

Many young people who engage in self-harm do not seek help from EDs, and those that do may experience negative attitudes from emergency service staff, which may be related to a knowledge and competency gap among staff as to the best way of providing optimal care [22]. Staff working in these types of stressful environments face elevated risk of fatigue and eventual burnout which can influence their ability to empathise yet they are often the key person in the young person's journey from admission to discharge.

Despite the 2001 World Health Organization global campaign to change negative public perceptions of mental health and the 2009 *Time to Change* challenge to tackle discrimination, stigma towards those with a mental illness remains a problem. Attitudes to mental ill-health range from empathetic to prejudicial coupled with limited knowledge of lived experiences. Mental ill-health is heterogeneous, and many of us do not know what it is like to experience a mental health condition first-hand. Emergency personnel who have experience of mental illness through a loved one or themselves are more likely to be tolerant of someone in a mental health crisis.

Police are often first on scene when a person is experiencing a mental health crisis and act as gatekeepers to the emergency care services. Historically police response and management of mental health crises have come under scrutiny, with deaths in custody, overuse of sections within the Mental Health Act (1983, 2007) [23] specifically s135 and s136 and use of excess force and arrest. Figures suggest a rise of 28% in incidents related to mental health between 2014 and 2018 with police feeling overstretched and lacking the skillset required to manage mental health crises, and the UK Government has pledged £2.3 billion to enhance mental health services by 2023/2024, to relieve the pressure on police [24].

Studies suggest that emergency medical staff often feel that mental health incidents involving low-level care and treatment or drug or alcohol misuse divert resources away from what is considered 'real' medical emergencies [25]. Reasons include working in a high-pressured role with limited time, labour and resources and limited mental health knowledge and awareness. Therefore, the onus is placed on universities to integrate better mental health education into their undergraduate courses, for purposes of awareness and skills to deal appropriately with patients in a mental health crisis.

The power imbalance between the patient and emergency personnel is real, whether those involved are aware, and perceptions may be determined by prejudged notions. The type of journey a CYP experiences through emergency care can depend on many factors such as their age, frequency of use of emergency services (the revolving door of mental health care) and complexities that ultimately shape the attitudes of emergency personnel. CYP who attend EDs for mental health issues, often feel they are left to the bottom of the list and their concerns are not taken seriously. However, factors such as environment, the perspective of the CYP and/or family and the confidence and/or knowledge/expertise of the ED practitioners can influence and evaluate changes in attitudes.

10 Care Pathways

The case study below depicts a typical scenario and the subsequent care pathway that may arise following a young person's admission to an ED.

10.1 Case Study: Ellie

10.1.1 Admission to an Emergency Department

Background

Ellie is a 15-year-old girl who presents to her local ED following an alleged overdose of 50 paracetamol tablets. She is irritable and uncooperative and doesn't want her mother to be involved in the assessment. Ellie has a 2-year history of co-existing oppositional behaviours, and she socialises with much older girls in the neighbourhood. She has become attached to the mother of one of the girls. Ellie also states that her parents are disinterested in her and never around. Furthermore, Ellie has an older boyfriend (aged 19) whom she met online, and her mother is very unhappy about this relationship and won't let her see him. Ellie says that she wants to live with her friend's mum as she is nice and spends time talking to her. She often goes there instead of going to school. Ellie says her mother is angry with her and doesn't believe that she has taken an overdose. She is refusing to have bloods taken and now wants to leave the ED. Her mother is sat in the waiting area.

Risk Assessment

It is extremely important for the assessing practitioner to persuade Ellie to have a risk assessment and explain to her that she would be interviewed alone first, then her mother will be interviewed separately, and, finally, to conclude the psychosocial assessment will be conducted, and they will then both be seen together. This is important as it allows both to have their say away from each other and then the plan can be shared with them both. The risk assessment should also include identification of protective factors, and the assessment should be shared with both parties. The assessing practitioner should follow the NICE guidelines on self-harm [26] for assessing risk.

It is very important to assess Ellie's capacity to consent and her understanding of being at risk of serious permanent injury from having no treatment for the paracetamol overdose. She would be viewed as currently being of significant risk, and the assessor would be required to involve her mother as Ellie is classed as a minor under the Mental Capacity Act/Mental Health Act (Mental Capacity (Amendment) Act, 2019; MHA, 1983 revised 2007) [27]. Additionally, her mother would also need to be assessed to ascertain whether she is capable to make decisions that are in the best interest of her daughter. If Ellie's mother is considered able (and gives appropriate consent), ED staff would be required to check paracetamol blood levels and commence treatment, if levels indicated. Any such treatment would have to take place on a paediatric ward as Ellie is under 16 years of age. As Ellie is under age and as her life may be at risk, her mother has parental responsibility, and confidentiality can be broken to safeguard Ellie under the zone of parental responsibility.

10.1.2 Post-initial Assessment at the ED

Second CAMHS Interview
Ellie is persuaded to have the blood test and to be admitted to the children's ward to undergo treatment as her paracetamol levels indicated the need to administer Parvolex. Post-medical treatment Ellie is seen by CAMHS for a further assessment. At interview she states that her mother has a drinking problem. She says also that she is scared of her own boyfriend and additionally admits to being sexually active with him. Again, she says she wants to live with her friend's mum. She knows her mother is angry with her and she can't tell her that she is scared of her boyfriend. She still wants to continue to see him, and she can't do that if she lives with her mother. She implies that she will take another overdose if she is made to go home. Conversely, her mother explains to the CAMHS practitioner that most of what Ellie says is not true, particularly in relation to how Ellie portrays her.

Management and Discharge
This type of scenario can be difficult to manage, and the assessing practitioner needs to be mindful that Ellie states her mother is abusing alcohol and that she is being sexually exploited by a 19-year-old-boy. She certainly meets 'child in need' criteria [28] which allocates duties to parents, social services, courts and other agencies to ensure children are safeguarded in this instance requiring urgent referral to social services prior to discharge from the paediatric ward. Social services may infer that she is not safe to go home post-discharge and would seek alternative accommodation. CAMHS and social services need to involve Ellie's mother in a discussion regarding safe discharge. Both services need to work together to agree the plan and share this with all concerned along with a rationale as to why this course of action is being taken. If Ellie were to abscond, the police would be alerted and any care planning meetings could include school staff. Certainly, the relationship she has with her friend's mother needs to be understood, and there may be further exploration of her relationship with her boyfriend, an adult.

The above case study illustrates a pathway, charting progress from admission to discharge for a young person entering the healthcare system. This type of assessment can be extremely sensitive and complex and requires involvement from a variety of professionals, significant adults and family. Effective and transparent communication can go some way towards alleviating the young person's distress. Further information on potential care pathways is described in the NICE guidelines for the long-term management of self-harm [29] which provides a web-based interactive flowchart of care pathways for different situations including:

- Initial management of self-harm by ambulance staff
- Management of self-harm in the ED

- Medical and surgical management of self-harm in the ED
- Psychosocial assessment of self-harm in the ED

In addition to these generic pathway choices and to ensure that all agencies and providers involved in care provision know their roles along a journey of care, integrated care pathways (ICPs) should be developed for each and every person entering the healthcare system. It is important that the person-specific ICP is communicated and made clear to the patient involved. The ICP should be tailored to the person and their needs and should be evidence-based and, importantly, person-centred. It should be designed so that it is clear to service users, their carers, and the multidisciplinary and multiagency care providers what should be expected at any stage of the journey through the healthcare system. Additionally, assessment of ICPs can be used to develop services and improve the patient's experience of the healthcare system, by comparing what was actually delivered to the patient compared to what the ICP had envisaged. Fragmented and disorganised care pathways can hinder the recovery of CYP, and poor communication can place a wedge in the therapeutic relationship between professionals, CYP and their families/carers. Despite integrated care being a central feature in the NHS Long-term Plan, there is a concern this is a finance-driven approach [30].

There are many examples of model ICPs which have been produced by various agencies and care providers and which can be used to inform how an ICP for a specific patient can be produced. Some are detailed and guide the assessor and others are subject to autonomy. A few examples exist in the following examples. The *Children and Young People's Health Partnership (CYPHP) Evelina London Model of Care* described as an innovative approach was developed by frontline practitioners, stakeholders, carers and health service commissioners. It integrates physical and mental health care and primary and secondary healthcare and attempts to address the social context of the family and strives to improve the wider determinants of health [31]. The *CYPHP* model has undergone an extensive research study in two large, highly populated boroughs in London; early indication suggests the innovative model is meeting the health needs of the population [32].

The *Cambridge University Hospital NHS Foundation Trust* assessment of CYP (under 18 years old) assesses the risks of the CYP to themselves in relation to self-harm and suicidal ideation and the risk to staff. There are five categories of questioning; 'issues to be explored through questioning', 'background, observations and behaviours', 'nursing assessment', 'suicide risk screen' and 'clinical assessment' which are set against a caveat of low, medium, and high risks, and actions are to be taken according to the risk at the time of presentation. The *University Hospitals Bristol* Children's ED uses a mental health assessment matrix, which has a similar framework to the one used by *Cambridge University Hospital*, yet it requests information on drug and alcohol consumption and has a clear designed formulation action plan. This formulation risk assessment plan sets out clear directions for the ED staff to follow, dependent on the level of risk. The *Manchester University NHS Foundation Trust* triage pathway clearly identifies that all CYP presenting at ED must be subject to a CAMHS assessment before they are discharged. The documentation identifies both physical and mental health concerns and key questions around suicidal ideation [33].

The following four principles are taken from the Department of Health Child and Adolescent Mental Health Services – A Service Model (2012) [34]:

- *Early Intervention* (services will work with family and carers).
- *CYP centred and family focussed* (families/carers and CYP actively involved in decisions – and will receive personalised care).
- *Help the CYP be the best they can be* (Staff will work with CYP to build on their strengths).
- *Integrated approach* (staff will ensure services will work together and that CYP/families/carers receive a consistent approach from all professionals working with them).

Mental health provision for CYP remains under-resourced, and emergency personnel would benefit from improved training or guidance to provide the appropriate and timely care, amidst increasing attendances to EDs. Despite ICPs shown in the CYPHP model, assessments are not evidence-based. The RCEM recommends that a risk assessment be completed by an appropriately trained mental health professional with CAMHS training to determine the care pathway.

The rise in mental health crises means that the health landscape of ED care provision continues to evolve at pace, across the four nations. Yet, government policies and Trust care pathways set impossible standards for ED personnel to achieve even when there has been considerable input from the emergency practitioner community. Standards require CYP to be assessed in a timely fashion, yet such timeframes are frequently breached, due to factors such as lack of provisions, resources, educational tools and an increasing need for support. ED personnel who treat CYP during a mental health crisis acknowledge that timely and quality treatment is difficult to achieve. The Mental Health Crisis Care Concordat is a welcome feature; however, there is still a long way to go to reach appropriate levels, and more input is needed to support quality improvement and service development.

11   Communication

As the above case study demonstrates, admission to a paediatric ward can cause anxiety for the young person and their families. Clinicians should develop a rapport to minimise misunderstandings and to allow the young person to open up about feelings. This can present significant challenges, and novice practitioners may be anxious about saying or doing the wrong thing, making a situation worse. Sometimes, as is the case with Ellie, responding accurately is a skill and practitioners need to seek clarification to help create some space for thoughts and demonstrate your wish to understand and care about her perspective on things.

Confidentiality is a key issue that needs to be addressed at the outset. To explain that any potential risks to self or others must be shared on a need-to-know basis and be flexible and responsive to the young person ensuring they are at the centre of the decisions. It is important not to pathologise normal emotions and reactions [35]. Being appraised as attention seeking can negatively impact on communication. Person-centred care is crucial, and this is now recognised across services as being a key ambition to optimising care for young people and their families. Practitioners need to be non-judgemental, empathetic and respectful, ensuring that the young person's views are prioritised and that they are empowered to make decisions about their care. Provision of person-centred care enables the young person to maintain their dignity and autonomy in the crisis.

The impact that self-harm can have on parents is substantial, and often the young person's perceptions of the event differ. Additionally, parents can feel the blame, yet they are often part of the solution particularly around having capacity to keep the young person safe. Being able to communicate effectively whilst balancing the therapeutic relationship with the young person can be a challenge. The global increase in self-harm among young people and the recent constraints due to the pandemic raises questions related to the availability and utility of resources to support both the young person and their family. Often their experiences can be omitted from their narratives and service provision. Self-harm can be a way of resolving conflict whilst conversely craving for care; therefore, space needs to be created for such cathartic expression. Table 1 provides a helpful list of 'Do's and Don'ts' suggested by service users with lived experience obtained during clinical practice by one of the authors [36].

The process of obtaining information is an important aspect of the care pathway yet can be a contentious issue for the CYP and their families/carers. The process by which information is retrieved is both arduous and time-consuming. The exchange of information is often requested on multiple occasions, by different personnel and each time the CYP and their family/carers are asked to provide dialogue and answer the same questions put forward to them. This process can be both frustrating and seem irrelevant and offer no timely solutions. It is important to highlight that emergency personnel ought to move past their own awkwardness and discomfort to frame questions openly and develop safety seeking behaviour in a timely fashion, especially in relation to suicidal attempts. Evidence-based assessments and care

Table 1 Young peoples' perspectives of attitudes and behaviour of professionals

Positive interventions	Avoid
• Be kind and non-judgemental	• Asking me how I am feeling on a scale of 1 to 10
• Be honest even if I do not want to hear it	• Pretending you know how I am feeling
	• Bringing your own issues into things
• Listen to what I am saying	• Diagnosing me!
• Be honest but above all be fun	• Using jargon
• Respect my rights for privacy	• Talking over me or about me when I am there
• Talk about other things besides my problem	• Getting frustrated when you cannot fix things
	• Saying 'superficial' or 'cry for help'
• Give me a sense of hope	• Faking sympathy or using your own personal strategies
• Discuss achievements	
• Allow me a safe place to be myself	• Being scared or frightened of me

pathways could support the emergency personnel, as could mental health and CAMHS training, to provide a more streamlined healthcare system.

12   Conclusion

The current emergency services system requires adjustment to work towards a more integrated system of response. For the system to work, emergency personnel need to work together to offer a timely support mechanism for the service user and their families/carers; and professionals need to be verse on what services are available in the locality: both NHS and local charitable organisations. In Liverpool, UK, there are over 150 charitable organisations dedicated to mental health services alone.

Emergency personnel may benefit the care process if they were to explore the wider issues: social determinants of health and factors that precipitate and perpetuate illness in so many CYP. Approaches should be integrated and child-friendly, recognise their needs and support them in a positive and tailored way.

Learning Points
- Make a list of ten communication qualities you possess when talking with CYP in mental health crisis and consider how, as an emergency practitioner, you might improve communication between the child, parent and referral services.
- Consider how emergency practitioners might offer a more integrated referral service to counter the negative effects of CYP mental health crisis.
- Identify the correct information in your department for community referral services to support CYP and their families.

Resources Available to Emergency Personnel
- NICE Guidance www.nice.org.uk/guidance
- Royal College of Psychiatry www.rcpsych.ac.uk
- Thrive, The AFC-Tavistock Model for CAMHS www.ucl.ac.uk/ebpu/docs/publication_files/New_THRIVE
- Quality Network for Community CAMHS (QNCC) www.qncc.org.uk
- Royal College of Psychiatry Leaflets for Young People www.rcpsych.ac.uk
- Young Minds www.youngminds.org.uk

References

1. Kessler RC, Amminger GP, Aguilar-Gaxiola S, Alonso J, Lee S, Ustün TB. Age of onset of mental disorders: a review of recent literature. Curr Opin Psych. 2007;20(4):359–64. https://www.ncbi.nlm.nih.gov/pmc/articles/PMC1925038/.   https://doi.org/10.1097/YCO.0b013e32816ebc8c
2. Department of Health. Future in Mind. Promoting, protecting and improving our children and young people's mental health and wellbeing. [Internet]. 2015 [cited 2021 Feb 12]. https://assets.publishing.service.gov.uk/government/uploads/system/uploads/attachment_data/file/414024/Childrens_Mental_Health.pdf

3. NHS Wales. Together for children and young people: framework for action. [Internet]. 2015 [cited 2021 Feb 12]. http://www.wales.nhs.uk/documents/Framework%20For%20Action.pdf

4. Scottish Government. Getting it right for every child (GIRFEC). [Internet]. 2006 [cited 2021 Feb 26]. https://www.gov.scot/policies/girfec/principles-and-values/#:~:text=Getting%20 it%20right%20for%20every%20child%20%28GIRFEC%29%20is,predict%20if%20or%20 when%20they%20might%20need%20support

5. Scottish Government. Mental health strategy 2017-2027. [Internet]. 2017 [cited 2021 Feb 26]. https://www.gov.scot/publications/mental-health-strategy-2017-2027/

6. Northern Ireland Commissioner for Children and Young People (NICCY). Still waiting. A Rights Based Review of Mental Health Services and Support for Children and Young People in Northern Ireland. [Internet]. 2018 [cited 2021 Feb 26]. https://www.niccy.org/media/3114/ niccy-still-waiting-report-sept-18-web.pdf

7. Northern Ireland Commissioner for Children and Young People (NICCY). Still waiting: status update report 2019. [Internet] 2019 [cited 2021 Feb 27]. https://www.niccy.org/ publications/2019/october/10/still-waiting-status-update-report/

8. NHS Digital. Health Survey for England 2018 [NS]. [Internet] 2018 [cited 2021 Jan 25]. https:// digital.nhs.uk/data-and-information/publications/statistical/health-survey-for-england/2018

9. Department of Health. Every child matters. [Internet] 2008 [cited 2021 Jan 27]. https:// assets.publishing.service.gov.uk/government/uploads/system/uploads/attachment_data/ file/272064/5860.pdf

10. HM Government. Working together to safeguard children. A guide to interagency working. [Internet] 2018 [cited 2021 Feb 26]. https://assets.publishing.service.gov.uk/government/ uploads/system/uploads/attachment_data/file/942454/Working_together_to_safeguard_chil- dren_inter_agency_guidance.pdf

11. NHS England. Achieving better access to 24/7 urgent and emergency mental health care. [Internet] 2016 [cited 2021 Feb 13]. https://www.england.nhs.uk/wp-content/uploads/2016/11/ lmhs-guidance.pdf

12. World Health Organization. Adolescent mental health. [Internet] 2012 [cited 2021 May 2]. https://www.who.int/news-room/fact-sheets/detail/adolescent-mental-health

13. Poutler D, Baig B, Cooney M, Cornick S. Child and adolescent mental health services: a case study in confused priorities. HSJ. 2018. Nov 23. https://www.hsj.co.uk/comment/child-and- adolescent-mental-health-services-a-case-study-in-confused-priorities/7023882.article

14. Royal College of Emergency Medicine. Mental Health in Emergency Departments. A tool- kit for improving care. [Internet] 2019 [cited 2021 Feb 26]. https://www.rcem.ac.uk/docs/ RCEM%20Guidance/Mental%20Health%20Toolkit%202019%20-%20Final%20.pdf

15. NHS England. New Care Models: Vanguards - developing a blueprint for the future of NHS and care service. [Internet] 2016 [cited 2021 May 15]. https://www.england.nhs.uk/wpcontent/ uploads/2015/11/new_care_models.pdf

16. NHS Long-term plan. [Internet] 2019 [cited 2021 May 15]. https://www.longtermplan.nhs.uk/

17. NICE. NICE impact children and young people's healthcare. [Internet] 2020 [cited 2021 Jul 2]. https://www.nice.org.uk/Media/Default/About/what-we-do/Into-practice/measuring-uptake/ children-young-people-impact-report/nice-impact-children-young-people-healthcare.pdf

18. Office for Health Improvement & Disparities. Children and Young People's Mental Health and Wellbeing. [Internet] 2019 [cited 2021 Jun 4]. https://fingertips.phe.org.uk/profile-group/ mental-health/profile/cypmh

19. YoungMinds [Internet]. 2018 [cited 2021 Jun 4]. https://youngminds.org.uk/about-us/media- centre/press-releases/ae-attendances-by-young-people-with-psychiatric-conditions-almost- doubled-in-five-years-new-figures/

20. Health London Partnership. Children and young people and mental health crisis care. [Internet]. 2020 [cited 2021 Jun 4]. https://www.healthylondon.org/our-work/crisis-care/ children-young-people-mental-health-crisis-care/

21. Her Majesty's Inspectorate of Constabulary and Fire and Rescue Services. Policing and Mental Health: Picking Up the Pieces. [Internet]. 2018 [cited 2021 Jun 7]. https://www.jus-

ticeinspectorates.gov.uk/hmicfrs/wp-content/uploads/policing-and-mental-health-picking-up-the-pieces.pdf

22. Byrne SJ, Bellairs-Walsh I, Rice SM, Bendall S, Lamblin M, Boubis E, McGregor B, O'Keefe M, Robinson J. A qualitative account of young people's experiences seeking care from emergency departments for self-harm. Int J Environ Res Public Health. 2021;18(6):2892. https://pubmed.ncbi.nlm.nih.gov/33808995/. https://doi.org/10.3390/ijerph18062892

23. Mental Health Act. 1983, as amended 2007. [Internet] 2007 [cited 2021 Aug 21]. https://www.legislation.gov.uk/ukpga/2007/12/contents

24. Jones L. Police dealing with more mental health incidents. BBC. [Internet] 2019 [cited 2021 Aug 22]. https://www.bbc.co.uk/news/uk-49317060

25. McCann TV, Savic M, Ferguson N, Bosley E, Smith K, Roberts L, et al. Paramedics' perceptions of their scope of practice in caring for patients with non-medical emergency-related mental health and/or alcohol and other drug problems: a qualitative study. PLoS One. 2018;13(12):e0208391. https://doi.org/10.1371/journal.pone.0208391.

26. NICE. NICE impact mental health. [Internet] 2020 [cited 2021 Mar 9]. https://www.nice.org.uk/Media/Default/About/what-we-do/Into-practice/measuring-uptake/children-young-people-impact-report/nice-impact-children-young-people-healthcare.pdf

27. Mental Capacity Act. 2005. [Internet] 2005 [cited 2021 Mar 9]. https://www.legislation.gov.uk/ukpga/2005/9/contents

28. Children Act. 2004. [Internet] 2004 [cited 2021 Mar 9]. https://www.legislation.gov.uk/ukpga/2004/31/contents

29. NICE. Self-harm in over 8s: long-term management. Clinical guideline CG133. [Internet] 2011 [cited 2021 Mar 9]. https://www.nice.org.uk/guidance/cg133

30. Royal College of Paediatrics and Child Health. Integrated care systems in Workforce development England – consultation response. [Internet] 2019 [cited 2021 Aug 21]. https://www.rcpch.ac.uk/resources/integrated-care-systems-workforce-development-england-consultation-response

31. Children and Young People's Health Partnership. Helping children and young people to be healthy, happy, and well. [Internet] 2019 [cited 2021 Aug 21]. https://www.cyphp.org/

32. Lingam R, Forman J, Newham J, Cousens S, Satherley R-M, El Sherbiny M, Wolfe I. The Children and Young people's Health Partnership (CYPHP) Evelina London Model of Care: an opportunistic cluster randomised trial to assess child health outcomes, healthcare quality, and health service use Int J Integr Care. 2019;19(4):381. https://pubmed.ncbi.nlm.nih.gov/31481366/. https://doi.org/10.5334/ijic.s3381

33. The Royal College of Emergency Medicine. Mental health in emergency departments. A toolkit for improving care. [Internet] 2019 [cited 2021 Aug 21]. https://www.rcem.ac.uk/docs/RCEM%20Guidance/Mental%20Health%20Toolkit%202019%20-%20Final%20.pdf

34. Family Support Northern Ireland. Working together: A pathway for children and young people through CAMHS. [Internet] 2018 [cited 2021 May 9]. https://www.familysupportni.gov.uk/Content/uploads/userUploads/CAMHS-Pathway.pdf

35. McCance T, McCormack B, Dewing J. An exploration of person centeredness in practice. Online J Issues Nursing. 2011; 16(2):1. https://pubmed.ncbi.nlm.nih.gov/22088150/

36. Trainor G. Self-harm in young people: risk factors, assessment and treatment interventions. A CPD resource. Nurs Child Young People. 2020;33:25. https://doi.org/10.7748/ncyp.2020.e1281.

Older People Mental Health

Deborah Goode, Vidar Melby, and Assumpta Ryan

1   Introduction

This chapter focuses on the older person and mental health within the emergency medical services care pathway. Mental health is defined as '…a state of well-being in which an individual realizes his or her own abilities, can cope with the normal stresses of life, can work productively and is able to make a contribution to his or her community' ([1], p. 38). Every person has a mental health need, whether it is a case of stress and anxiety before an exam or a diagnosed functional or organic mental illness. For the purpose of this chapter, the term mental health need/s will refer to a person who has a mental health problem or disorder including dementia [2] and an older person referred to as someone aged 65 years or older.

The number of people within the general population at present who experience mental health issues is increasing, with 1,028,081 people having contact with adult mental health services in England [3]. Mental health needs can be described as organic (affects memory and other functions associated with old age) and functional (where there is no evidence of organic disturbance). The Royal College of Psychiatrists [4] highlighted the relevance of growing numbers in 2005, stating that 60% of patients over 65 years of age admitted to general hospitals have, or will develop, a mental health problem such as dementia, delirium, or depression. By 2017 the WHO [5] reported worldwide figures of around 15% of people who were over 60 and had a mental health disorder. Methods of collecting data differ around the world, with differing definitions of old age; however, one key point

D. Goode (✉)
University of Ulster, Belfast, Northern Ireland
e-mail: d.goode@ulster.ac.uk

V. Melby · A. Ryan
University of Ulster, Derry/Londonderry, Northern Ireland
e-mail: v.melby@ulster.ac.uk; aa.ryan@ulster.ac.uk

© The Author(s), under exclusive license to Springer Nature Switzerland AG 2023
T. Scott (ed.), *Mental Health: Intervention Skills for the Emergency Services*,
https://doi.org/10.1007/978-3-031-20347-3_9

remains: a delay in seeking help can affect the outcome of treatment. There are also challenges around the availability and adequacy of mental health treatment [6].

According to the World Health Organization [7], people are living longer and also living more years with good health. Global life expectancy rose from 66.8 years in the year 2000 to 73.3 years in 2019. Presently, 13.5% of the world's population is over 60; by 2030, it is projected that one in six people will be 60 years of age or older, with this figure rising to two billion by 2050 [8]. This means that the current proportion of the global population over 60 years of age will almost double to 22%.

The literature on people presenting with mental health needs in the emergency department (ED) is substantial; however, reported statistics vary for a variety of reasons. Up to 5% of patients who present at ED have a psychiatric disorder, and a further 20–30% present with physical and psychiatric disorders [9]. Whilst 5.3% of patients who presented to ED (aged 18–65 years) had a mental health issue [10], ED visits for older people with mental health disorders accounted for 27.3% of attendances, with 51.2% being admitted [11]. Other studies report that the figure for admission for this group of people is even higher at 84.7% [12], possibly due to a reluctance by older people to seek help. Any delay could lead to their condition worsening which would then require additional, more complex treatment and admission to hospital.

When older people with mental health needs attend ED and other acute care settings, they have a higher risk of poor outcomes than the general older population. In a large-scale observational examination of older people in the ED ($n = 2252$) within 13 EDs in seven nations (Australia, Belgium, Canada, Germany, Iceland, India and Sweden) [13], results showed:

- Increased vulnerability (compared with the general population under 75 years of age) with 67% of the older people being dependent on someone else for one or more activity of daily living.
- 26% of respondents had evidence of memory loss.
- 48% had a geriatric syndrome (age-related decline including issues such as multiple health conditions, issues with mental function, frailty, disability and malnutrition) prior to attending the ED and this figure rose to 78% on presentation to ED.

These figures were consistent across the seven nations in the study. High levels of delirium (27%) and dementia (47%) were also reported in a population of patients ($n = 249$) over 70 years old who presented at hospital due to an emergency [14]. So, to dispel a myth, despite the increasing numbers of older people, they are not the highest users of ED. From 2010 to 2020, those aged 65 years and over presented in smaller percentages (19.2–22%) than the 15–34 (26.8–30.1%) or 35–64 (30.4–31.3) age groups [3].

2 Environment for Care

Provision of care within the pre-hospital and ED pathway has inherent challenges. Pre-hospital staff frequently work alone (if they are a single paramedic/rapid responder) or with a colleague in a vehicle that supports care for a variety of patients with differing conditions. They must be able to assess, treat and transport the person to another level of care (if that is possible and appropriate). Often, they attend people who due to impairment provide only a very limited physical and mental health history, and they provide care in the home or community environment. In the ED, similar challenges are faced by the team. Staff are unaware of who will present to the department until they arrive (unless alerted by the ambulance team), what they are attending for or what treatment will be needed. Planning and preparation within the department requires knowledge of how the whole hospital is functioning (ED waiting times, bed availability, through to admission and discharge) and an awareness of the readiness of the ED facility and staff. These challenges in both the pre-hospital and ED environments can impact on the quality of care provided for older people with mental health needs.

Some of these challenges were discussed in a modified scoping study on the effect of the ED culture in relation to the care given to older adults [15]. ED is viewed as the 'front door of the hospital' with the promise that no one will be turned away from the department but assessed and prioritised based on triage. The number of patients who attend the ED can mean that it appears as a noisy, busy, complex and stressful environment. Some patients report that they cannot identify staff and found identification badges hard to read. The values and beliefs held by ED staff demonstrated that the ED was an environment for treating urgent cases; however, it was also viewed as a safe place where anyone could find help and support. Time was an urgent issue in ED, with older people needing more assessment and treatment, this time was seen to take up resources that were needed for others, perceived to be of a higher priority. Older people were viewed as a lower priority which meant longer waiting times associated with complex care needs. ED staff reported that the needs of older people who were not critically ill would have been better met in the community setting.

Some of these challenges were also presented in an examination of the literature surrounding the provision of person-centredness in the ED environment [15]. The environment was portrayed as one where a highly complex range of skills were needed to attend to the wide variety of patients; however, the focus of care was on medical, technical and emergency tasks. Caring for patients who were not 'in need' of ED care such as minor complaints, end of life and mental health issues was reported as conflicting with the ED culture of caring for urgent and emergency cases. The priority for ED staff was to move patients through the department as quickly and efficiently as possible; this was often not possible due to numbers and types of patients attending as well as lack of beds in the hospital system. This certainly would be the case for older people with mental health needs attending the ED as they often require more complex assessments and admission to hospital for further care [12].

3   Why Older People Attend ED

The reasons for attending ED are varied, with the majority of older people 'walking in' with urgent treatment needs (Table 1). Older people with a mental health issue attend ED possibly due to a lack of access to a GP, loneliness and social isolation. Patterns of attendance are evenly spread throughout the year, with an increase in the winter months, notably December and January. Older people with mental health needs who attend ED are more likely to be female and attend on a Monday and usually in the morning.

In a study of older people ($n = 74,766$) in one region of the UK who attended ED, shortness of breath/pulmonary embolism (9.1%) was the main reason for attending. Other common reasons were falls (8.5%), chest pain (7.2%) and limb injury (7.1%) [12]. Older people had several needs that required consideration when being discharged from ED ranging from aftercare issues, medications, unresolved medical problems and health risk. These issues also impacted on repeat attendances at ED by older people for social, physical, mental and comorbid problems [16].

Table 1   Main reasons older people attend ED [16]

Cardiovascular problems (acute and chronic) 10–41%
Musculoskeletal problems were reported as minor or major trauma and issues associated with poor mobility (76% of the older people in one study had fallen)
Intestinal disorders, urinary tract (plus kidney disease and failure), gastrointestinal tract, pain and metabolic disorders on 13–32%
Older people also had adverse drug reactions that caused problems with organ function and reaction (metabolic 20%, neurological 17% and cardiovascular 17% in nature)
Dermatological problems (including skin cancer) were reported in the review to account for 2–33% of presentations to ED by older people, whilst neurological conditions varied from 2 to 18%
Accidents also were a major reason for older people attending ED with 60% occurring in their home

4   Policy Impacting on Older Person Emergency Care

The WHO stated that despite the worldwide increasing numbers of older people in society, there remains a low level of training for all staff within the area of gerontology and education and training, a low priority focus for governments [17]. NICE [18, 19] recommend training for health and social care practitioners so they may recognise and respond to many of the medical and other support needs of older people. The need for health and social care (HSC) practitioners to recognise deterioration in an older person and to refer onward to the most appropriate support service was also highlighted [18, 19]. The Royal College of Psychiatrists (RCP) recommend that more health and social care professionals are trained in general and specialist areas of care provision to older people with mental health needs [20]. There has certainly been an increased focus on mental health within the NHS over the past decade with guidance documents produced in England for improving access [19], assessment of the frail older person that includes a geriatric assessment [21] and new ways of working [22, 23]. In Northern Ireland, the Bamford *Review of Mental Health and Learning Disability* resulted in an action plan from the Northern Ireland Executive which aimed to begin to improve health and social care in Northern Ireland alongside the *Transforming Your Care* review [24]. However, a review for Action Mental Health [25] found that there were still gaps in service provision, mainly due to lack of funding. This is consistent with the findings from EMS staff who reported a lack of 'joined-up-care' for older people with mental health needs and who were frustrated by the lack of continuity in community care provision and support for carers. Integrated urgent care key performance indicators (IUC) are outlined by NHS England [23] to link the care provided to older people in the community before they are taken to ED for treatment. This may also assist in earlier recognition of areas that need assessment and support.

Caring for older people with mental health needs in pre-hospital and acute care areas has been a source of question and concern worldwide. Following evidence of lack of investment in mental health care and ageist attitudes toward people with mental health needs, recommendations for the provision of equitable, high-quality mental health care for older people were provided by the Mental Health Foundation [26]. Acute care liaison and support should be available from mental health practitioners, with staff trained in the recognition and treatment of both physical and mental health needs for older people to provide treatment that is fair and equitable. The Equality Act [27] brought together many different areas of legislation to protect the older person from unfair or discriminatory service provision in the UK; however, Northern Ireland (NI) still operates under several different orders. Personalised care and support at the level of need, rather than of age, are one of the key recommendations for planning this service. Integrated physical care and mental health care, with equal levels of priority, were promoted by the government as the only way forward [28]. However, this 'ageless service' concerned the then Chief Medical Officer Dame Sally Davies [29], because the need to care for an older person with physical, mental and social difficulties requires specialist education and training and could be compromised by a move to a generic service. The Urgent and Emergency Care (UEC) service proposes to deliver all age 24/7 mental health crisis care by 23/24 [30].

5   The Complexity of Older Person Presentations

5.1   Associated Multimorbidities and Polypharmacy

An older person with mental health needs can often have diagnosed and undiagnosed comorbidities. The use of the medical model for assessment and curative care for this group of patients and their families and carers assesses immediate need and does not provide care for other needs [31]. The use of shared, consistent multidisciplinary team (MDT) care in hospital, care homes and in the community is the preferred goal [32], and it is suggested that skills in mental health and palliative and supportive care for EMS staff are developed alongside acute medical and rehabilitation care.

The complexity of caring for a physically unwell older person who also has mental health needs was acknowledged by Goldberg et al. [33], who reported that patients with mental health problems who were admitted to hospital as an emergency had functional needs associated with incontinence (47%), mobility (49%) and feeding (49%). Cognitive impairment was present in 79% of the sample. These patients were more likely to be agitated and apathetic, have motor behaviour problems and be delirious than those in the sample who did not have cognitive impairment. Numbers were high on admission to acute areas, but with the older people aged 75 years and older, the rate of cognitive impairment was around 50%, with a third of these older people having no previously known dementia or delirium [34].

5.2   Co- or Multimorbidity

Comorbidity refers to the person having more than one health condition, which may explain the impact it has on the person through illness or disease. Multimorbidity is usually when two or more chronic diseases co-occur. Table 2 highlights four areas that should be assessed during examination.

Multimorbidity can lead to geriatric syndromes and disability. Geriatric syndromes represent changes that can occur in the body in conjunction with the ageing process, and they can lead to the development of conditions that cause multiple organ impairment in older people [36]. Some of these are cognitive impairment, frailty, sarcopenia, falls, urinary incontinence and pressure injury. The presence of 'geriatric syndrome' in older patients was reported in a large-scale international multisite study (Australia, Belgium, Canada, Germany, Iceland, India and Sweden)

Table 2 Four areas should be assessed when examining co- or multimorbidity [35]

1. The nature and definition/classification of the health condition (diseases, disorders, conditions, illnesses or health problems)
2. Relative importance of the conditions as they occur with others (complications or interactions, chronic or acute)
3. Chronology of the presentation of the conditions (time span and sequence of occurrence)
4. Morbidity burden and patient complexity (how these conditions impact the physiological dysfunction/frailty/severity as well as cultural, behavioural, socioeconomic and environmental characteristics)

[13]. The rate of cognitive impairment was reported as 26% in the ED compared to 20% prior to the illness. Delirium was suggested in 16% of the patients as there was an acute change in mental state. Sixty percent of the older people who attended ED were admitted into acute care wards. This study shows that these older people are mostly dependent and frail and have both physical and cognitive functioning decline. Over 75% of patients had at least one geriatric syndrome, and this pattern was consistent across the developed nations [13].

5.3 How Comorbidities Impact on the Older Person

The nature and degree of comorbidity makes the care for older people who also have mental health needs/issues much more complex. The older person may not be able to recall an accurate history of the recent illness or trauma. It is important that all healthcare professionals have the knowledge, skill and ability to assess these complex needs. The resources required to provide an appropriate care package are often unavailable in the acute care and community areas. The projected rise in numbers of older people with mental health needs using the National Health Service (NHS) will have implications for how general acute hospital wards are staffed, with an emphasis on the environment, training and expertise of EMS staff and partnership with the family. Consideration should be given to the complexity and interaction of pharmacological, cognitive, physical and social needs of older people presenting to EDs as these are associated with greater risks of falls, fractures and delirium [37].

5.4 Impact of Polypharmacy

Polypharmacy is the term used to describe the use of multiple medicines for one person that occurs because the person has one or more conditions and is prescribed medication/s to treat them resulting in the accumulation and use of multiple medications. Polypharmacy (6–9 prescriptions over 3 months) is associated with adverse health outcomes in older people after attending ED [38]. Reasons could be associated with the lack of expertise in polypharmacy by prescribers and the potential reactions, interactions and adverse consequences in the older person. An indication

Table 3 International variation in reported instances of polypharmacy [38]

USA had the lowest prevalence at 10.7% (Gu 2010)
17 European countries in the (SHARE) database figures were between 26.3 and 39% (Midão et al. 2018)
Sweden 44% (Morin et al. 2018)
In Korea 86.4% of older adults aged 65 and over (Kim 2014) with similar figures reported in Taiwan 83.5% (Chan et al. 2009)

of the prevalence of polypharmacy is shown in Table 3; however, figures vary internationally as differing ages and definitions of polypharmacy were used.

5.5 The Complexity of Delirium and Dementia

Delirium is defined by the WHO ICD-10 [39] as:

> An aetiologically nonspecific organic cerebral syndrome characterized by concurrent disturbances of consciousness and attention, perception, thinking, memory, psychomotor behaviour, emotion, and the sleep-wake schedule. The duration is variable and the degree of severity ranges from mild to very severe.

It is a condition that develops over hours or days that results in an acute deterioration of the person's mental functioning. Delirium is often linked with poor outcomes in older people and can be caused by an acute illness or infection, drugs, surgery or trauma. The RCEM developed an online learning package entitled 'Delirium in the Elderly', which outlines the need for an accurate assessment including history taking and examination to diagnose and treat delirium (The Royal [40]. Delirium is a common medical emergency (20% of acute medical patients) and common risk factors to consider are outlined in Table 4.

The nature of the complexity and combination of possible presentations emphasise the importance of knowing that effective treatment is based on the early identification and treatment of the cause of the condition. Dementia on the other hand is a progressive and terminal condition. The Royal College of Nursing [43] explain that:

> The term dementia is used to describe a range of conditions which affect the brain and result in an impairment of the person's function. The person may experience memory loss, problems with communication, impaired reasoning and difficulties with daily living skills. (p. 5)

Many of the common symptoms of dementia can also be present in people who have delirium (e.g. short term memory loss, difficulties in communication, orientation and perception, hallucinations and psychological changes), adding further complexity to the care of people with mental health needs. Screening for dementia of all older people over 65 in the ED is suggested, as approximately 50% of older people who attend ED who do not have their dementia diagnosed are at high risk of functional decline [44].

Table 4 Risk factors for delirium within a medical assessment

NICE include risk factors for delirium within the medical assessment [41]
• Age 65 years of age or older
• Past or present cognitive impairment and/or dementia
• Current hip fracture (affects up to 50% of cases)
• Severe illness
SIGN also add the following risk factors [42]
• Frailty https://www.bgs.org.uk/resources/silver-book-ii-frailty
• Multiple comorbidity
• Male gender
• Sensory impairment
• History of depression
• History of delirium
• Alcohol misuse

6   Communication, Capacity and Consent (Mental Health Act 2005)

The use of effective methods of working with older people with cognitive and sensory impairment is a special skill set, and effective communication can reduce errors, increase safety and improve patient outcomes. There is a need for training for all MDT members on effective communication with the older person with mental health needs, including the effect the physical environment (including sensory stimulation) can have, especially someone living with dementia. This training should include the impact on the family and how they can be involved in care. The *Silver Book II* [45] reflects the importance and relevance of this issue within their suggestions for training and development in knowledge, skills and attitudes.

Communication can become more complex in emergency settings when considering the person's capacity to make decisions regarding their own care. Consent to treatment is a legal requirement in healthcare and a professional requirement in ensuring best practice, evidence-informed assessment, clinical decision-making and accountability. Legislation differs across the four countries within the UK. The RCEM [46] outlined best practice guidelines in emergency medicine to comply with the Mental Capacity Act (MCA), 2005 [47]. The MCA aims to protect and empower people who may lack the mental or cognitive ability (capacity) to make decisions about their own care and treatment. It should be assumed that anyone over 16 has capacity unless proven otherwise.

Assessing capacity:

- Does the person have a cognitive impairment (due to alcohol, drug use, illness, injury, learning disability)?
- Does this impairment mean that a specific decision about their care cannot be taken at this moment in time (as capacity can fluctuate)?

According to the Mental Capacity Act 2005 [47], to be able to decide, the person must be able to:

- Understand all of the information about the decision they are being asked to make.
- Be able to retain this information.
- Comprehend the information in an appropriate manner and weigh it up in the decision-making process.
- Communicate that decision by any means.

Best-interest decisions are those which are made for the person who lacks capacity to decide about their care and should be the least restrictive alternative when considering their rights and freedoms. When making a best-interest decision, the healthcare professional should:

- Identify all the relevant circumstances.
- Discuss with the person and identify their views, feelings, wishes, beliefs and values on the topic under discussion.
- Involve the person in the decision-making.
- Avoid discrimination.
- Consider if the person may regain capacity. The decision may be able to be postponed.
- Discuss with next of kin/family/named individuals or anyone caring for them.
- Consult with anyone who was appointed under Lasting Power of Attorney/ Enduring Power of Attorney, or anyone appointed by the Court of Protection.

In some cases, the person may have restrictions placed upon them known as deprivation of liberty (DOL). This is when the person no longer has the capacity to make decisions about their own care; decisions are made for them about keeping the person safe and ensuring correct medical treatment. Each person must be judged individually and strict DOL safeguards must be employed.

7   Early Assessment and Improvements in Patient Flow for the Older Person

In the emergency pathway early assessment is vital. To be able to holistically assess and treat this patient group within a short period of time requires a high level of competence in both physical and mental health conditions [26]. The primary focus of EMS staff is the culture of 'fixing problems' that are usually physically orientated and that mental health assessment and care are of a secondary priority. The RCEM [48] emphasises that:

> The Core Principle of Mental Health in the Emergency Department: A patient presenting to ED with either a physical or mental health need should have access to ED staff that understand and can address their condition, and access to appropriate specialist services, regardless of their postcode, GP or time of arrival (P2).

The RCEM [48] outlines mental health audit standards for individual patients and the ED, whereby a mental health triage assessment should be completed when older people present to the ED and should include a capacity assessment if required. The recommended assessment tool in the ED, according to NICE [49], is the Australian Mental Health Triage Tool, alongside the use of an appropriate proforma that includes mental health details and a safe discharge plan. Changing the initial method of triage to 'initial senior assessment and treatment' model improved quality of care (timely and appropriate diagnosis, early treatment and intervention, improved transit time in the department) as well as the experience by the older person [50].

Since 2008, the USA has seen the emergence of EDs with a focus on older people (geriatric EDs). Guidance was approved in a collaboration between the American College of Emergency Physicians, the American Geriatrics Society, Emergency Nurses Association and the Society for Academic Emergency Medicine in 2013 [51]. Recommendations included the following:

- Staff should be appropriately educated and experienced (medical director and nurse manager, specialist physicians and nurses, pharmacists, social workers and consultants in old age).
- Follow-up care should include discharge protocols with clear information including presenting complaint, tests and results, treatment completed and response, medical summary, discharge diagnosis, new and existing prescriptions and follow-up plan. Links should be maintained with the community, nursing and residential sectors.
- Educational programme for all staff.
- Quality improvement programme to include data on numbers of attendances, admission rate, readmission rate, deaths, suspected abuse or neglect, transfers to higher level of care, return visits within 72 hrs, at-risk screening tool, follow-up from discharge, falls, catheters, medication management and delirium.
- Equipment and supplies including appropriate layout, lighting and noise.
- Policies and procedures including triage, assessment and screening.

Similar older person's EDs (OPED) were set up in the UK to integrate many of these recommendations the first being Norfolk and Norwich University Hospitals NHS Foundation Trust in 2016.

---

8   The Older Person's Emergency Care Journey

Pre-hospital emergency care and the ED can be distressing and frightening for older people (with or without mental health needs). When the older person has to call the ambulance or attend the ED because of an illness, these feelings of apprehension and fear escalate. Being ill at home or in the community setting can often be the first step in the older person's journey and contact with pre-hospital staff, and transport by ambulance can be the first of many care transitions for them. In the ED, the noisy, busy, complex and stressful environment can impact on the older person who has mental health needs. In these care environments, the attitudes, values and beliefs of the staff are important, as well as the knowledge and skills to deliver safe, effective, timely, dignified and compassionate care for the patient and family.

It is recognised that attending ED is a stressful experience that can cause fear and anxiety. Older people want professional, competent care, including information about what is happening and how long they will wait. They have concerns about the ED design and how the department functions and have variable levels of tolerance or ability to cope with the situation [52, 53]. Cetin-Sahin et al. [54] reported on the older person's experience in ED [54] and areas of concern focused on:

- The ability to meet physical needs (comfort, equipment to support mobility, access to help when needed, as well as access to food and fluids).
- Family members want to be contacted, to be physically with the older person and to be involved or participate in the care.
- Transitional care needs. When the older person leaves the ED, they want to understand that the health problem is resolved. They need discharge information including medication and future care. Safe transport from the ED and arrangement for follow-up or home care services is also deemed important.

The patient experience is also a major concern for the RCEM [55] who published their best practice guideline which includes 50 care standards for emergency care. The checklist includes themes about the environment, the ED team and the patient pathway and caring for older patients and patients with complex needs. These themes are emphasised in the RCEM Mental Health in ED toolkit [48], which emphasises a suitable area for assessment, observation and one-to-one nursing. Additionally, educational developments include competencies for older people and mental health care in the National Curriculum and Competency Framework for Emergency Nursing [56]. The College of Paramedics include mental health in their latest curriculum guidance document [57]. It was also evident in the literature that more specialist knowledge and skills are required to care for older people (with and without mental health needs) in acute settings [13, 16, 26, 58, 59].

Older people with mental health needs have poorer outcomes of care when compared to the same age group who do not have any mental health issues [60–62]. Older adults, in general, spend a long time waiting in EDs (300.6 min), and those who also have a mental health issue waited even longer (344.7 min) [12]. In other quality indicators, the care is unequal in terms of a longer length of stay, increased reattending, increased risk of falling, reduction in activities of daily living (ADL) and way they are perceived and treated by some healthcare staff. The rates of readmission and hospitalisation are also high which require appropriate care planning, discharge and continuity of care as older people are more likely to be discharged to a long-term care facility [31]. Increased functional decline in both physical and mental realms is evident as well as a marked increase in mortality, both whilst in hospital and following discharge [63].

9   Involving the Family

Involving the family in care of an older person attending the ED can assist in communication and explanations. Experiences of family and those who care for older people with mental health needs during admission to acute care in the UK were examined [64]. Carers expressed several core problems during the period their relative was in the acute care hospital. The carers reported a 'disruption from their normal routine' that could apply to both their routine and the routine of the older person being cared for. They coped with this problem by trying to establish some level of control over the situation through effective communication. This helped the carer to cope as they felt they had a form of protection over their relative by taking the role of advocate, often making evaluations of the care provided and the ward environment. They also coped with the situation by supporting hospital staff in caring for their relative (and fill the gaps in care). Relatives also became stressed when they felt they could not trust the staff to provide good, personalised care for their relative. Quality of care was a prominent issue, relating to the way the patient and relative were communicated within a triadic manner, especially with the skill of listening. Healthcare professionals should recognise the vital role of the family as being the expert in the care of their family member, someone who can support care delivery and become a partner in care [64]. John's Campaign began in 2014 to support people who live with dementia to be supported in hospital by their family members [65].

The experience of the person and family members in ED can relate directly to their perceptions of the quality of medical and nursing care, how long they have to wait and the ability to be diagnosed (availability of diagnostic testing and equipment). Regular communication including explanations of challenging situations is an essential part of the involvement of the family in ED care [66]. Caring for the family in a time of crisis or illness by responding to their need for honest, clear, information and proximity to their family member was reported as a method of developing ways of coping with the stress and anxiety of the crisis [67].

10   Dignity, Choice and Person-Centred Care

Person-centredness has become a central tenet of health and social care, particularly over the past decade and in particular in relation to older people [68, 69]. The focus on improved standards of care delivery since the Francis Report [70] emphasised the relevance of holistic and collaborative care that places the person at the centre of their care. The research literature on person-centred care in the pre-hospital and emergency care environment is sparse; indeed, in 2016, no papers were identified on person-centredness as a concept in ED [15] though the term 'patient-centred' may reveal a few since that date. McCormack and McCance propose that to achieve person-centred outcomes a number of components need to be in place [68, 69].

Professional competency and good interpersonal skills are essential when assessing and treating an older person with mental health needs in the pre-hospital and emergency care environment. The care environment should encourage effective staff relationships, a supportive organisational structure and a suitable physical environment. If these components are in place, the care processes of providing holistic care, shared decision-making and working with patient's beliefs and values and engagement can move toward achieving person-centred outcomes of satisfaction with care, involvement in care, feeling of well-being and creation of a therapeutic culture [69]. Themes in the ED literature suggest that the environment and culture of ED could be problematic in achieving person-centred outcomes for older people with mental health needs [15, 71, 72].

The National Institute for Health and Care Excellence (NICE) [18] recommends that all patients have the right to a high standard of coordinated, safe and effective person-centred care that meets their needs. However, to deliver care that is based on individual needs, there must be a thorough assessment. The older person and their carer should be involved in the care planning with clear and unambiguous language used to ensure understanding. Support provided must progress toward achieving their care needs and be reviewed regularly. Care and support should be given in a respectful way that promotes trust and dignity. Holistic person-centred care should be provided to the highest standard and the independence and advocacy of the person promoted [73]. Unfortunately, this is not always the case, and unmet mental health needs of older people are discussed in an aptly titled report *'Hidden in Plain Sight'* [74]. It is widely accepted that older people have physical and mental comorbidity; however, almost 40% of mental health trusts in England do not have a strategy or policy to support comorbidity in the older person. This is concerning as the projected 12% rise in numbers of older people in the UK by 2021 will undoubtedly increase the pressure on the NHS [74]. Despite assessment guides such as that produced by the Social Care Institute for Excellence [75] to assist in the assessment of mental health needs of older people, the issue of inequality of care remains unresolved. The challenge is not only faced in the UK and Ireland, but with the pressure of assessing and treating ageing patients with complex needs, it has become an international concern. Many challenges are faced in primary care, with each of the ten countries (Australia, Canada, Germany, the Netherlands, New Zealand, Norway, Sweden, Switzerland, the UK and the USA) involved in the aforementioned study facing the same issues [76]. They were all ill-prepared and had variable experiences in coordinating care between primary and secondary care sectors. This is of particular relevance to pre-hospital emergency care and the interface with emergency care settings.

11   End-of-Life Care

It is widely accepted that the provision of quality end-of-life care is central to effective and culturally sensitive person-centred care [77]. End-of-life care within the pre-hospital and ED setting can be challenging due to the often unexpected or

Table 5 End-of-life care for adults in the emergency department

All staff should receive regular training in all aspects of end-of-life care
Patients and their families should be involved, wherever possible, in end-of-life care decisions. All discussions should be documented, with details of who took part in the discussions
ED doctors should endeavour to determine what end-of-life care plans have already been made by having access to electronic end-of-life care registers and by asking the patient and their family
Discussions regarding patient treatment preferences should be communicated to GPs, care homes and inpatient teams to enable continuity of care and end-of-life care planning
If a patient is at the end-of-life, it may be appropriate to set a ceiling of treatment in the ED
Establishing a 'do not attempt cardiopulmonary resuscitation' order (DNACPR) should not always limit other care given. A statement of planned active care should also be documented where appropriate including what care should and should not be provided
Patients nearing the end-of-life should have a resuscitation decision made before leaving the ED, and this should be appropriately documented
All DNACPR decisions should be discussed with the patient's family and the patient unless the patient is unable to understand the decision or unless it is thought the discussion will cause physical or psychological harm to the patient, family or carers
Clinicians should be trained and able to commence medicines for symptom control. A checklist or other end-of-life care documentation may be useful so that all necessary aspects of care are considered
Opportunities for organ and tissue donation should be considered as a usual part of end-of-life care in the ED
All EDs should have procedures for dealing with sudden death including clinical governance review
All EDs should have adequate facilities for dealing with bereaved relatives

traumatic events that occurred and the impact this can have on the family. The ED environment is not a quiet or private area for a person at the end-of-life and their family. Some palliative care areas use a butterfly symbol to identify the person is at the end of their life; other areas use a three stranded white spiral (Irish Hospice Foundation) to convey compassion. This can be useful for the whole team within ED to be aware of what is happening in the department. Best practice guidance has been developed by RCEM [78] to assist staff in these situations including regular training and support (Table 5).

12   Interagency Collaboration

The quality of care for older people with mental health needs in the pre-hospital and acute and emergency care areas has been a source of question and concern world-wide. Following evidence of lack of investment in mental health care and ageist attitudes toward people with mental health needs, recommendations for the provision of equitable, high-quality mental health care for older people were provided by the Mental Health Foundation [26]. They suggest that acute care liaison and support should be available from mental health practitioners, with hospital staff trained to recognise and manage both physical and mental health needs of older people.

Several National Health Service (NHS) commissioning priorities have been presented [22], and there is a need to develop an integrated response to improve the management of patients who have both mental and physical health needs. They recognised the extent to which mental health can be a comorbidity for many people, often causing an increase in the risk of poor health outcomes. Several changes to current practice were suggested including improved assessment and recording of mental health conditions. They assert that there is a lack of robust evidence on health outcomes and suggest that by improving care coordination, the impact on the quality of life for older people with multiple comorbidities can improve significantly. The area of effective urgent and emergency care also requires an integrated approach involving hospital, community, primary and ambulance services, with the government committed to reducing the inequality in care provided to people with mental health and learning disability by 2020. Such support and care are often accessed in the pre-hospital setting and EDs, and this care should be effective and based on clear roles, protocols and responsibility with appropriate liaison with mental health services [22, 79, 80].

The National Confidential Enquiry into Patient Outcome and Death (NCEPOD) *Treat As One: Bridging The Gap Between Mental And Physical Healthcare In General Hospitals* report makes several principal recommendations [81]:

- Liaison psychiatry services should be part of the MDT and should be fully integrated into acute hospitals.
- Staff who interact with patients (including security, clerical and clinical) should have training in managing people with mental health needs.
- Mental health conditions should be assessed and documented alongside any physical conditions that may have brought the person to hospital. There should be clear and concise plans documented at time of the assessment.
- National guidelines for the management of people with mental health conditions admitted to acute hospitals should be developed.
- Improved sharing of medical notes between mental health and acute hospitals is necessary.

Interagency collaboration and integrated care pathways for older people (including older people with mental health needs) are suggested; however, there are cultural, institutional, economical and educational components that must be established [82]. To date the evidence for coping with increased demand or improved efficiency through the use of integrated care methods is not available. There is, however, some evidence that the use of an integrated care system may increase patient satisfaction and access to services [83].

13   Conclusion

The chapter has presented information on mental health, older people and the emergency pathway. It is clear that education and training of EMS staff to competently assess and provide care for older people and their families is of paramount importance in maintaining dignity and compassion for this population and for future planning of EMS care. Legislation and guidance will continue to focus this care on person-centred practices. Development of OPEDs appear to improve satisfaction with treatment and could be developed with interagency collaboration to provide a more individualised approach to care of the older person with mental health needs.

Learning Points
- Write a few sentences about how you may enhance your knowledge, attitude and skills to provide high quality person-centred care to the vulnerable older person with mental health needs.
- Consider what changes you could make in the emergency care pathway and the EMS environment to reduce stress and anxiety experienced by older people with mental health needs.
- Explain how you would assess mental capacity to ensure that older people with mental health needs are centre stage in decision-making about their care.

References

1. World Health Organization. Promoting mental health. Concepts, emerging evidence, practice. Geneva: WHO; 2004.
2. Sartorius N. Mental health needs, 2015: changes of concepts and consequences. Psychiatry Clin Neurosci. 2015;69:509–11.
3. National Health Service (NHS) Digital. Hospital Accident & Emergency Activity 2019–20. London: NHS Digital; 2020. https://digital.nhs.uk/data-and-information/publications/statistical/hospital-accident%2D%2Demergency-activity/2019-20/summary-reports
4. Royal College of Psychiatrists. Who cares wins. London: The Royal College of Psychiatrists. 2005. http://www.rcpsych.ac.uk/PDF/WhoCaresWins.pdf
5. World Health Organization. Integrated care for older people guidelines on community-level interventions to manage declines in intrinsic capacity. Geneva: WHO; 2017.
6. Bunting BP, Murphy SD, O'Neill SM, Ferry FR. Lifetime prevalence of mental health disorders and delay in treatment following initial onset: evidence from the Northern Ireland study of health and stress. Psychol Med. 2012;42:1727–39. https://doi.org/10.1017/S0033291711002510.
7. World Health Organization. World health statistics. Geneva: WHO; 2021. https://cdn.who.int/media/docs/default-source/gho-documents/world-health-statistic-reports/2021/whs-2021_20may.pdf?sfvrsn=55c7c6f2_18
8. World Health Organization. Decade of healthy aging. Geneva: WHO; 2021. https://www.who.int/publications/i/item/9789240023307
9. Bolton J. Psychiatry in the emergency department. Psychiatry. 2009;8(6):185–8.
10. Shafiei T, Gaynor N, Farrell G. The characteristics, management and outcomes of people identified with mental health issues in an emergency department, Melbourne, Australia. J Psychiatr Ment Health Nurs. 2011;18:9–16.
11. Hakenewerth AM, Tintinalli JE, Waller AE, Ising A. Emergency department visits by older adults with mental illness in North Carolina. Western. J Emerg Med. 2015;XVI(7):1142–5.
12. Goode D, Slater P, Ryan A, Melby V. A comparison of the time spent in emergency departments by older adults with and without mental health needs. Adv Emerg Nurs J. 2021;43(2):145–61. https://doi.org/10.1097/TME.0000000000000350.
13. Gray LC, Peel NM, Andrew P, Costa AP, Burkett E, Dey AB, Jonsson PV, Lakhan P, Ljunggren G, Sjostrand F, Swoboda W, Wellens NIH, Hirdes J. Profiles of older patients in the emergency department: findings from the interRAI multinational emergency department study. Ann Emerg Med. 2013;62(5):467–74.

14. Whittamore KH, Goldberg SE, Gladman JRF, Bradshaw LE, Jones RG, Harwood RH. The diagnosis, prevalence, and outcome of delirium in a cohort of older people with mental health problems on general hospital wards. Int J Geriatric Psychiatry. 2014;29(1):32–40. https://doi.org/10.1002/gps.3961.

15. McConnell D, McCance T, Melby V. Review: exploring person-centredness in emergency departments: a literature review. Int Emerg Nurs. 2016;26:38–46. https://doi.org/10.1016/j.ienj.2015.10.001.

16. Šteinmiller J, Routasalo P, Suominen T. Older people in the emergency department: a literature review. Int J Older People Nursing. 2015;10(4):284–305.

17. World Health Organization. World report on ageing and health. Geneva: WHO; 2015.

18. National Institute for Health and Care Excellence. Older people with social care needs and multiple long-term conditions. London: NICE; 2015.

19. National Institute for Health and Care Excellence. Achieving better access to 24/7 urgent and emergency mental health care – part 2: implementing the evidence-based treatment pathway for urgent and emergency liaison mental health services for adults and older adults – guidance. London: NICE; 2016.

20. Royal College of Psychiatrists. The need to tackle age discrimination in mental health. A compendium of evidence. London: RCP; 2009. https://www.rcpsych.ac.uk/pdf/Royal%20College%20of%20Psychiatrists%20-%20The%20Need%20to%20Tackle%20Age%20Discrimination%20in%20Mental%20Health%20Services%20-%20Oct09.pdf

21. NHS England. Safe, compassionate care for frail older people using an integrated care pathway: practical guidance for commissioners, providers and nursing, medical and allied health professional leaders. London: NHS; 2014.

22. Naylor C, Imison C, Addicott R, Buck D, Goodwin N, Harrison T, Ross S, Sonola L, Tian Y, Curry N. Transforming our health care system. Ten priorities for commissioners. London: The King's Fund; 2015.

23. NHS England. Next steps on the NHS five year forward view. London: NHS England; 2017. www.england.nhs.uk/publication/next-steps-on-the-NHS-five-year-forward-view/

24. Department of Health, Social Services and Public Safety Northern Ireland. Transforming your care. A review of health and social care in Northern Ireland. Belfast: DHSSPSNI; 2011. http://www.dhsspsni.gov.uk/transforming-your-care-review-of-hsc-ni-final-report.pdf

25. Wilson G, Montgomery L, Houston S, Davidson G, Harper C, Faulkner L. Regress? React? Resolve? An evaluation of mental health service provision in Northern Ireland. Belfast: Action Mental Health & Queen's University Belfast; 2015.

26. Mental Health Foundation. All things being equal. Age equality in mental health care for older people in England. London: Mental Health Foundation; 2009.

27. Equality Act. London: HMSO. 2010. https://www.gov.uk/guidance/equality-act-2010-guidance#equalities-act-2010-legislation

28. Department of Health. Closing the gap: priorities for essential change in mental health. London: DH; 2014.

29. Davies SC. Annual report of the chief medical officer. Public mental health priorities: investing in the evidence. London: Department of Health; 2014.

30. National Health Service. NHS mental health implementation plan 2019/20–2023/24. London: NHS; 2019. https://www.longtermplan.nhs.uk/wp-content/uploads/2019/07/nhs-mental-health-implementation-plan-2019-20-2023-24.pdf

31. Bradshaw LE, Goldberg SE, Lewis SA, Whittamore K, Gladman JRF, Jones RG, Harwood RH. Six-month outcomes following an emergency hospital admission for older adults with co-morbid mental health problems indicate complexity of care needs. Age Ageing. 2013;42(5):582–8.

32. Department of Health. The Government's mandate to NHS England for 2016–17. London: DH; 2017.

33. Goldberg SE, Whittamore KH, Harwood RH, Bradshaw LE, Gladman JRF, Jones RG. The prevalence of mental health problems among older adults admitted as an emergency to a general hospital. Age Ageing. 2012;41(1):80–6.

34. Pendlebury ST, Klaus SP, Mather M, De Brito M, Wharton RM. Routine cognitive screening in older patients admitted to acute medicine: abbreviated mental test score (AMTS) and subjective memory complaint versus montreal cognitive assessment and IQCODE. Age Ageing. 2015;44(6):1000–5.

35. Valderas JM, Starfield B, Sibbald B, Salisbury C, Roland M. Defining comorbidity: implications for understanding health and health services. Ann Fam Med. 2009;7(4):357–63. https://doi.org/10.1370/afm.983.

36. Cheung JTK, Yu R, Wu Z, Wong SYS, Woo J. Geriatric syndromes, multimorbidity, and disability overlap and increase healthcare use among older Chinese. BMC Geriatr. 2018;18:147. https://doi.org/10.1186/s12877-018-0840-1.

37. Benavidez G, Garrido M, Frakt A. Transforming emergency departments to better care for elderly patients. JAMA Forum Archive. 2018;12 https://doi.org/10.1001/jamahealthforum.2018.0036.

38. Salvi F, Rossi L, Lattanzio F, Cherubini A. Is polypharmacy an independent risk factor for adverse outcomes after an emergency department visit? Intern Emerg Med. 2017;12(2):213–20. https://doi.org/10.1007/s11739-016-1451-5.

39. World Health Organization. The ICD-10 classification of mental and behavioural disorder. Diagnostic criteria for research; 2016. https://icd.who.int/browse10/2016/en#!/F00-F09

40. The Royal College of Emergency Medicine. Delirium in the elderly. London: RCEM; 2020. https://www.rcemlearning.co.uk/reference/delirium-in-the-elderly/#1568885316660-7e4ed5cb-6911

41. National Institute for Health and Care Excellence. Delirium: prevention, diagnosis, and management. London: NICE; 2020.

42. Scottish Intercollegiate Guidelines Network (SIGN). Risk reduction and management of delirium. A national clinical guideline. Edinburgh: NHS Scotland; 2019. https://www.sign.ac.uk/media/1423/sign157.pdf

43. Royal College of Nursing (RCN). Commitment to care of people living with dementia. SPACE principles. London: RCN; 2019.

44. Grimmer K, Beaton K, Kumar S, Hendry K, Moss J, Hillier S, Forward J, Gordge L. Estimating the risk of functional decline in the elderly after discharge from an Australian public tertiary hospital emergency department. Aust Health Rev. 2013;37(3):341–7.

45. British Geriatric Society. Silver Book II. Quality urgent care for Older people. BGS; 2021. https://www.bgs.org.uk/resources/resource-series/silver-book-ii

46. The Royal College of Emergency Medicine. The mental health act in emergency medicine practice. London: RCEM; 2017.

47. Department of Health. Mental capacity act. London: HMSO; 2005.

48. The Royal College of Emergency Medicine. Mental health in emergency departments toolkit. London: RCEM; 2021.

49. National Institute for Health and Care Excellence. Managing self-harm in emergency departments. London: NICE; 2021.

50. Ameh V, Nasir H, Ahmed S, Abassi A. Improving patient flow in an emergency department. Br J Health Manage. 2018;24(10):486–90.

51. The American College of Emergency Physicians, The American Geriatrics Society, Emergency Nurses Association, and the Society for Academic Emergency Medicine. Geriatric Emergency Department Guidelines. New York: ECEP/AGS/ENA/SAEM; 2013.

52. Bridges J. Listening makes sense: understanding the experiences of older people and relatives using urgent care services in England. London: City University; 2008.

53. Watson WT, Marshall ES, Fosbinder D. Elderly patients' perceptions of care in the emergency department. J Emerg Nurs. 1999;25(2):88–92.

54. Cetin-Sahin D, Ducharme F, McCusker J, Veillette N, Cossette S, Vu TTM, Vadeboncoeur A, Lachance PA, Mah R, Berthelot S. Experiences of an emergency department visit among older adults and their families: qualitative findings from a mixed-methods study. J Patient Experienc. 2020;7:346–56. https://doi.org/10.1177/2374373519837238.

55. The Royal College of Emergency Medicine. Emergency departments care. London: RCEM; 2017.

56. Royal College of Nursing. National curriculum and competency framework emergency nursing (level 1). London: RCN; 2017.
57. College of Paramedics. Paramedic curriculum guidance. 4th ed. Bridgewater: TCOP; 2017.
58. Bunn F, Dickinson A, Simpson C, Narayanan V, Humphrey D, Griffiths C, Martin W, Victor C. Preventing falls among older people with mental health problems: a systematic review. BMC Nurs. 2014;13(4):1–15. http://www.biomedcentral.com/1472-6955/13/4
59. Faulkner D, Law J. The 'unnecessary' use of emergency departments by older people: findings from hospital data, hospital staff and older people. Aust Health Rev. 2015;39(5):544–51.
60. Mather B, Roche M, Duffield C. Disparities in treatment of people with mental disorder in non-psychiatric hospitals: a review of the literature. Arch Psychiatr Nurs. 2014;28:80–6. https://doi.org/10.1016/j.apnu.2013.10.009.
61. Sampson EL, Leurent B, Blanchard MR, Jones L, King M. Survival of people with dementia after unplanned acute hospital admission: a prospective cohort study. Int J Geriatr Psychiatry. 2013;28(10):1015–22.
62. Schnitker L, Martin-Khan M, Beattie E, Jones RN, Gray L. Negative health outcomes and adverse events in older people attending emergency departments: a systematic review. Australas Emerg Nurs J. 2011;14:141–62.
63. Adams LY, Koop P, Quan H, Norris C. A population-based comparison of the use of acute healthcare services by older adults with and without mental illness diagnoses. J Psychiatr Ment Health Nurs. 2015;22:39–46.
64. Clissett P, Porock D, Harwood RH, Gladman JR. Experiences of family carers of older people with mental health problems in the acute general hospital: a qualitative study. J Adv Nurs. 2013;69(12):2707–16.
65. AgeUK. Implementing John's campaign. London: Age UK; 2016. https://www.ageuk.org.uk/contentassets/8e71b5353aa641739a7aa751e7ab0ec5/age-uk-john_s-campaign-guide.pdf
66. Salehi T, Nayeri ND, Mohammadi E, Mardani-Hamooleh M. Exploring patients' and family members' experiences of care in the emergency department. Emerg Nurse. 2020. https://doi.org/10.7748/en.2020.e2008. https://journals.rcni.com/emergency-nurse/evidence-and-practice/exploring-patients-and-family-members-experiences-of-care-in-the-emergency-department-en.2020.e2008/abs
67. Botes M, Langley G. The needs of families accompanying injured patients into the emergency department in a tertiary hospital in Gauteng. Curationis. 2016;39(1):a1567 ISSN: (Online) 2223-6279, (Print) 0379-857.
68. McCormack B, McCance T. Development of a framework for person-centred nursing. J Adv Nurs. 2006;56(5):472–9.
69. McCormack B, McCance T. Person–centred nursing theory and practice. Chichester: Wiley-Blackwell; 2010.
70. Francis R. Report of the mid Staffordshire NHS foundation trust public inquiry. London: The Stationery Office; 2013.
71. Marynowski-Traczyk D, Broadbent M. What are the experiences of emergency department nurses in caring for clients with a mental illness in the emergency department. Australas Emerg Nurs J. 2011;14(3):172–9. https://doi.org/10.1016/j.aenj.2011.05.003.
72. Wright ER, Linde B, Rau L, Gayman M, Viggiano T. The effect of organizational climate on the clinical care of patients with mental health problems. J Emerg Med. 2003;29(4):314–21.
73. Skar P, Bruce A, Sheets D. The organizational culture of emergency departments and the effect on care of older adults: a modified scoping study. Int Emerg Nurs. 2015;23(2):174–8.
74. Stickland N, Gentry T. Hidden in plain sight. The unmet mental health needs of older people. London: Age UK. 2016.
75. Social Care Institute for Excellence. NICE social care mental health guidance. https://www.skillsforcare.org.uk/Learning-development/social-work/Mental-health-social-work/NICE-social-care-mental-health-guidance.aspx
76. Osborn R, Moulds D, Schneider AC, Doty MM, Squires D, Sarnack DO. Primary care physicians in ten countries report challenges caring for patients with complex health needs. Health Aff. 2015;34(12) https://doi.org/10.1377/hlthaff.2015.1018.

77. Goode D, Black P, Lynch J. Person-centred end-of-life curriculum design in adult pre-registration undergraduate nurse education: a three-year longitudinal evaluation study. Nurse Educ Today. 2019;82:8–14. https://doi.org/10.1016/j.nedt.2019.07.009.
78. The Royal College of Emergency Medicine. End of life care for adults in the emergency department. London: RCEM; 2015.
79. Department of Health (and Concordat signatories). Mental health crisis care concordat – improving outcomes for people experiencing mental health crisis. London: DH. 2014.
80. Turner J, Bjarkoy M, Coleman P, Goodacre S, Knowles E, Mason S, Nichol J, O'Cathain A, O'Keeffe C, Wilson R. Building the evidence base in pre hospital urgent and emergency care. A review of research evidence and priorities for future research. University of Sheffield: Department of Health. 2010. https://www.sheffield.ac.uk/polopoly_fs/1.43655!/file/Evidence-base.pdf
81. National Confidential Enquiry into Patient Outcome and Death (NCEPOD). Treat as one bridging the gap between mental and physical healthcare in general hospitals. London: NCEPOD. 2017. https://www.ncepod.org.uk/2017mhgh.html
82. Harnett PJ, Kennelly S, Williams PA. 10 step framework to implement integrated care for older persons. Ageing Int. 2020;45:288–304. https://doi.org/10.1007/s12126-019-09349-7.
83. Baxter S, Johnson M, Chambers D, Sutton A, Goyder E, Booth A. The effects of integrated care: a systematic review of UK and international evidence. BMC Health Serv Res. 2018;18:350. https://doi.org/10.1186/s12913-018-3161-3.

Toxicology in Parasuicide

Karen Osinski

1   Introduction

Poisoning is an age-old phenomenon with Paracelsus declaring in the sixteenth century that the only difference between a therapeutic effect and a poisonous effect is the dose of the substance. The risk of harm from overdose generally relates to the substances involved and the therapeutic index profile attached to each substance. Therapeutic index refers to the relative safety of a drug by comparing the amount of drug required for a therapeutic effect with the amount of drug which will cause toxicity. Drugs with a broad therapeutic index may be relatively safe in overdose, whereas drugs with a narrow therapeutic range are much more hazardous in overdose (e.g. lithium, digoxin and phenytoin).

The most common mode of self-harm resulting in presentation to hospital is self-poisoning. Annually, in the UK there are approximately 160,000 NHS emergency department presentations attributed to poisoning, in addition to many more consultations at primary care and NHS advice services such as NHS 111, NHS 24 and NHS Direct [1]. There is significant mortality risk attached, with the World Health Organization estimating that around 800,000 people die as a result of suicide yearly [2]. There are five broad categories into which poisoning can be distributed:

- Accidental: most common in children
- Occupational: occurring in the context of employment
- Environmental: referring to exposure from chemicals in the air, water or food
- Recreational: usually ingestion of illicit substances

K. Osinski (✉)
Clinical Toxicology Advanced Nurse Practitioner, National Poisons Information Service,
Edinburgh, UK
e-mail: karen.osinski@nhslothian.scot.nhs.uk

© The Author(s), under exclusive license to Springer Nature
Switzerland AG 2023
T. Scott (ed.), *Mental Health: Intervention Skills for the Emergency Services*,
https://doi.org/10.1007/978-3-031-20347-3_10

- Deliberate or intentional: with the aim of self-harm or death

Additionally, poisoning may be a result of acute ingestions or may be due to chronic exposures. However, poisoning requiring referral to hospital is most commonly due to acute intentional overdose of pharmaceutical products, particularly in Western countries. A vital aspect of managing the patient post-overdose concerns the time interval. Clarification of time since overdose and staging of time passed allows practitioners to hypothesise the trajectory and plan for potential clinical developments. The first stage is always to determine what substances have been ingested, how much and at what time.

Patients presenting to the emergency department post-overdose are often emotionally distressed, intoxicated or acutely agitated on arrival to hospital. It can prove challenging to provide essential clinical care in these circumstances, but forming a therapeutic and empathic relationship is important to progress appropriate management of the physiological aspects of the overdose. This is an extremely sensitive time for both the patient and their family but can also impact on the practitioners involved.

2 Risk Assessment

It is essential to consider the twofold risks of the presentation. There is the potential for clinical harm from the overdose itself as well as the potential for further self-harm if the patient has ongoing suicidal or self-harming ideation. It is always helpful to conduct a risk assessment focussing on suicidality or thoughts of self-harm which involves asking some difficult questions. Keep in mind the priority is the patient's safety during what may be an incredibly stressful situation. The overdose may have been taken impulsively in response to life stressors, or it may have been a strategically planned event with attempts to conceal the act. These offer variable degrees of risk in themselves, and it is important to probe a little deeper to clarify risk of further self-harm. This is valuable in the acute presentation; however, all patients presenting post-overdose with self-harm or suicidal intent must be referred for a formal review by a psychiatry team prior to discharge from hospital.

To gauge level of risk, the practitioner should enquire into the intent of the overdose after clarification of substances taken and timings of overdose as follows:

- Was this a single ingestion?
- What time were the tablets taken?
- Was the overdose staggered?
- Taken over hours or days?

Consider asking 'What did you expect to happen when you took the overdose?' and if there was anything in particular that drove the act (triggers). It is also helpful to ascertain whether there are support networks in place or things that the person finds joy or safety in (protective factors) that may prevent a further attempt. Indeed, the patient may have experienced a relationship breakdown or bereavement that has triggered the act but may now feel regretful and can describe protective factors in family, friends, pets, career or hobbies. Conversely, the person may feel there was no particular trigger and that this event was an accumulation of long-standing issues and are now unable to provide any suggestions of hopefulness for the future. It is useful to ask *'Now that you are in hospital, how do you feel about what happened?'* Furthermore, asking about future plans following discharge from hospital is valuable in assessing risk. It may occur, despite carefully phrased questions, that the patient may refuse to answer, or major inconsistencies may arise. For example, the patient who has taken an impulsive overdose in the knowledge it was likely to be harmless may now report that they intend on 'doing it properly' by committing suicide on discharge. Alternatively, the patient who had been found by chance following a concealed and potentially fatal overdose may now appear bright and positive about the future. This may present a predicament for the practitioner, and many clinicians describe relying on intuition. Ultimately patients presenting post-self-harm should be observed closely with steps taken to minimise risk. It is pertinent to gently ask if the patient has any further medications or implements that could be used to self-harm (e.g. razors, ligatures) and request to remove these. Patients who present to emergency areas post-self-harm often report feeling marginalised by healthcare professionals [3]. It may be difficult for the patient to gain trust, particularly in emergency settings where practitioners may be unfamiliar to them; it is vital that practitioners remain nonjudgemental and empathic. To develop therapeutic relationships, we must dedicate time to create a safe environment to provide honest and empathic consultation and care.

3 Clinical Assessment

Patients may present asymptomatically, and it is vital to undertake clinical risk assessment considering potential or emerging harms, investigations required and management. Conversely, they may present very acutely unwell and in need of rapid initiation of antidotes or supportive care. It can be complicated to clarify the situation if the patient is intoxicated, acutely distressed, unconscious or reluctant to engage. It may be possible to piece together the history by means of witness accounts, collateral from family members regarding available substances in the home and from ambulance reports of evidence at the scene. Patients may display toxidromes, a term which describes a cluster of features (or syndrome) associated with different groups of drugs (examples shown in Table 1). Recognition of toxidromes may provide more evidence to guide clinical diagnosis. Specific toxidromes will be discussed in more detail further in this chapter when considering the most common poisoning presentations.

It often takes some degree of detective work to fully clarify the nature of the overdose. Once we have some understanding of the clinical situation, it is essential that practitioners know how to access the most comprehensive advice to ensure best possible outcomes.

Table 1 Examples of toxidromes

Toxidrome	Potential causative agents	Features
Anticholinergic	Atropine, tricyclic antidepressants, chlorpromazine, diphenhydramine	Hypertension, tachycardia, pyrexia, mydriasis, hot flushed skin, dry mouth, urinary retention, delirium, mumbling, seizures
Cholinergic	Organophosphates, carbamates	Miosis, profuse sweating, bronchial secretions, confusion, seizure, CNS depression
Opioid	Morphine, heroin, methadone, fentanyl	Bradycardia, hypotension, reduced respiratory rate, hypothermia, miosis, reduced bowel sounds, lethargy, drowsiness, coma
Sympathomimetic/serotonergic	Amphetamine, MDMA, selective serotonin reuptake inhibitors	Tachycardia, hypertension, tachypnoea, mydriasis, pyrexia, profuse sweating, agitation, paranoia, seizures
Sedative/hypnotic	Benzodiazepines, gabapentin, pregabalin	Hypotension, bradycardia, hypothermia, lethargy, drowsiness, coma

4 Poisons Advice

After clarifying the nature of the overdose, healthcare professionals dealing with poison exposures should *always* access TOXBASE®, the online clinical toxicology database. TOXBASE® is the UK source of the most robust and comprehensive information and management advice on over 21,000 substances ranging from organic compounds, household products, pharmaceutical medicines and drugs of abuse to the management of chemical incidents. This database is maintained by the National Poisons Information Service (NPIS) and provides healthcare professionals with global access to an up-to-date, accurate reference resource for advice on the features and management of the poisoned patient. All NHS facilities can register for free web access and 24-h enquiry service for individual advice on complex presentations (Box 1).

Box 1 National Poisons Information Service: Adapted from National Poisons Information Service [1]
Website details: www.toxbase.org
  24-h information for healthcare professionals: 0344 8920111
  Members of the public should contact NHS advice centres, e.g. NHS 24, NHS 111 or NHS direct or in Ireland contact NPIC
  TOXBASE admin: mail@toxbase.org
  NPIS: www.npis.org

Pre-hospital consultation of TOXBASE® is a particularly useful step in order to gauge toxic doses of ingested substances and whether or not the patient requires referral to hospital. For example, in the incidence of accidental ingestion of silica gel, this is considered a low toxicity substance and may be safely managed at home with advice to seek medical advice should symptoms develop. It is also possible that a patient requires referral to hospital following a modest overdose although asymptomatic as there is potential for emerging clinical features which would require management. For asymptomatic presentations, TOXBASE® provides guidance on minimum observation periods that should be fulfilled before the patient can be safely discharged home with advice to seek medical attention should symptoms develop. In hospital it is an invaluable tool for guiding the patient journey with the most up-to-date directions for care. If the presentation is complex or if more support is required, the team should contact NPIS directly. The NPIS is located over four NHS teaching hospitals in Birmingham, Newcastle, Cardiff and Edinburgh with links to consultant specialists in York and London. Their remit includes NHS education on poisoning therapies, public health surveillance and clinical toxicology research. However, the primary role of the NPIS is to provide 24-h poisons information to healthcare professionals via TOXBASE® access and telephone enquiries. Of interest, the majority of enquiries to NPIS relate to paracetamol poisoning, and this is reflected clinically in the volume of patients presenting to hospital post-paracetamol overdose. The following section examines the three main intentional overdose presentations in the UK: paracetamol, selective serotonin reuptake inhibitors (SSRIs) and tricyclic antidepressants (TCAs).

5   Paracetamol

Paracetamol is an analgesic and antipyretic available on prescription and as an over-the-counter product. Its easy access contributes to its regular use in overdose in the UK. Paracetamol is recognised as a very safe drug in therapeutic dosing; however, in overdose it can be fatal. Approximately 40% of all poisoning presentations are due to paracetamol overdose, which is the leading cause of acute liver failure in the UK.

5.1   Mechanism

In therapeutic dosing, paracetamol produces the toxic metabolite N-acetyl-para-benzoquinone imine (NAPQI) through oxidation via cytochrome P450 (CYP) enzymes in the liver. Glutathione stored in the liver quickly combines with NAPQI to form nontoxic cysteine or mercaptate conjugates which can be eliminated in urine. In overdose, however, it is believed that the glutathione stores are depleted by the overwhelming volume of NAPQI, thus allowing NAPQI to accumulate and bind to key cell components, setting in action a sequence of events leading to hepatocellular death [4]. The main goal in treating paracetamol poisoning is timely administration of an antidote in order to prevent this mechanism and reduce the likelihood of liver injury or failure.

5.2   Clinical Features

The early features of paracetamol poisoning are usually vague and may include nausea and vomiting. Those patients who have taken a significant overdose will go on to develop more serious features of hepatic impairment during the days following ingestion. It can be a relatively slow process and may (rarely) be accompanied by features of renal impairment. Right upper quadrant (or hepatic) tenderness can develop within 12-h. Clotting disorders may develop 3–6 days following ingestion as the liver becomes increasingly dysfunctional. Other features of progression towards liver failure include jaundice, encephalopathy, ascites, acidosis, spontaneous bruising and hypoglycaemia. In severe incidences headache has been noted as cerebral oedema occurs, raising intracranial pressure and resulting in reduced consciousness and brain stem coning. The rate at which fulminant liver failure ensues depends on the severity of overdose. In very severe poisoning, jaundice can develop within 24-h. Although the main feature of paracetamol poisoning is hepatic injury, in some rare cases, renal injury can occur in conjunction with hepatic failure or in isolation, presenting as loin pain, haematuria or proteinuria with an elevated serum creatinine.

5.3   Antidote

Acetylcysteine is the gold standard for treating paracetamol poisoning and has been used globally since the 1970s when it was found to drastically reduce mortality and hepatotoxicity rates if given within an ideal timeframe. Acetylcysteine is not only a precursor to cysteine which has antioxidant qualities; it also acts as a precursor to glutathione thus replenishing glutathione stores in order to conjugate with the toxic metabolite NAPQI, allowing safe elimination.

Acetylcysteine has generally been given as a 21-h intravenous treatment regimen. The total dose equals 300 mg/kg, comprising an initial bag of 150 mg/kg over 1-h, followed by a second bag of 50 mg/kg over 4-h and finally, a third bag of 100 mg/kg over 16-h. Following treatment with acetylcysteine, blood is analysed to monitor plasma paracetamol clearance and to check for alanine transaminase (ALT) elevation indicating hepatocyte injury and international normalised ratio (INR) rise which may indicate impaired liver function. However, acetylcysteine itself can cause a rise in INR and should be interpreted carefully. If necessary, according to criteria, additional infusions with acetylcysteine are commenced [1]. This infusion regimen, although extremely effective, is complex, with potential for drug miscalculations as well as dose-related anaphylactoid reactions during the highly concentrated first infusion.

5.4   Anaphylactoid Reactions

Dose-related vomiting and anaphylactoid reaction occur in up to 60% of patients in the initial treatment phase of acetylcysteine, which correspondingly leads to regimen interruption and refusal from 20% of patients [5]. Such reactions include flushing, urticaria, bronchospasm as well as nausea and vomiting. These symptoms can be managed by pausing the infusion and treating with antihistamine, antiemetic and salbutamol nebuliser in the instance of bronchospasm. It is vital to note that the infusion *can* be restarted and, indeed, *must* be restarted. These reactions are not true anaphylaxis although they are uncomfortable, and they are usually resolved by pausing the infusion alongside administration of the aforementioned medications. The infusion may be recommenced after half an hour and administered at half the original rate to facilitate tolerance. The second bag can then be infused at the advised rate.

5.5   SNAP Regimen

Many clinical areas, both nationally and internationally, now implement a novel regimen introduced following the Scottish and Newcastle Antiemetic Pre-treatment for Paracetamol Poisoning (SNAP) clinical trial [6]. This trial hypothesised that a 12-h two bag acetylcysteine course comprised of 100 mg/kg over 2-h followed by 200 mg/kg over 10-h could be designed as an alternative to the standard 21-h three bag regimen, while still providing the 300 mg/kg dose required for liver protection. The trial was conducted over 2 years, and a follow-up observational study concluded that the SNAP regimen produced fewer adverse reactions and had the same efficacy to prevent liver injury as the original regimen. Additionally, the shortened duration of therapy vastly improved rates of adherence to treatment.

5.6   Management

At the point of presentation to hospital, it must be determined whether or not acetylcysteine is required. Paracetamol poisoning is managed according to time of presentation post-ingestion and whether or not the ingestion was single or staggered/multiple. Paracetamol ingestions comprise three broad time categories: single acute ingestions, staggered and therapeutic excess, and each will be presented below. Single acute ingestions are further categorised into presentations at 0–8-h post-ingestion, 8–24-h and more than 24-h.

5.6.1   0–8-h Post-ingestion

The most straightforward scenario concerns the patient who presents early following a single acute ingestion (defined as an overdose taken within 1-h). In this scenario administration of activated charcoal should be considered in the first instance. Activated charcoal interferes with hydrolysis in the small intestine and actively absorbs many poisons within the gastric contents which limit toxic effects. It can effectively reduce the absorption of paracetamol if given within the first hour post-ingestion but can only be given if there are no airway concerns as there is risk of aspiration if the patient is drowsy. The next stage is to check a plasma paracetamol concentration at 4-h post-ingestion. This is vital to gain an accurate peak plasma level to determine whether or not a patient requires treatment. Urea and electrolytes (U&Es) must be analysed to assess renal function, as well as bicarbonate, liver function tests and INR to assess liver function and/or injury. Elevation in ALT or INR strongly suggests inconsistency with reported time of ingestion; therefore treatment would be indicated. Bicarbonate provides insight into possible developing acidosis in the instance of massive overdose. A full blood count is required as a baseline. For the patient presenting over 4-h from ingestion, the paracetamol concentration should be measured as soon as possible. Once obtained, this is plotted on the paracetamol nomogram found on TOXBASE® to deduce whether or not treatment is necessary (Fig. 1). If treatment is required, it is important to commence acetylcysteine as quickly as possible and within 8-h of ingestion to achieve the best possible protection.

If a patient presents early following a massive paracetamol ingestion confirmed by extreme plasma concentrations and evidence of mitochondrial dysfunction, specifically high lactate levels, metabolic acidosis or coma; haemodialysis may be warranted. However, due to timing, haemodialysis is inappropriate for the vast majority of patients who present following paracetamol overdose. If they present too early, acetylcysteine would be effective, and if they present too late, the remaining plasma paracetamol burden is too minor to justify invasive removal [7]. It is uncommon, yet entirely possible for the patient whose 4-h paracetamol level is over 700 to have a low bicarbonate indicating acidosis. In this instance blood gas analysis may reveal elevated lactate which would indicate some degree of organ dysfunction. These patients should be urgently discussed with the critical care team to consider urgent haemodialysis.

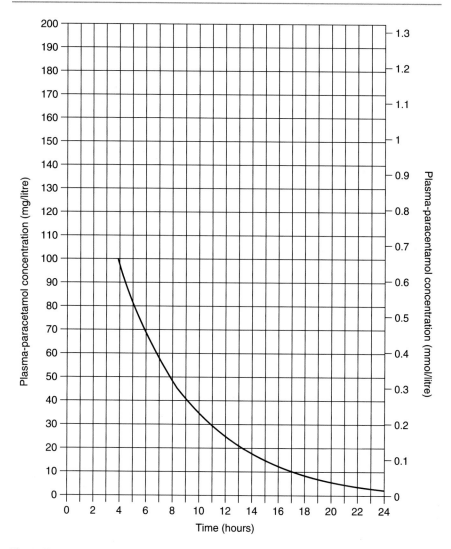

Fig. 1 Paracetamol treatment nomogram *for use only with paracetamol poisoning advice provided by www.toxbase.org. Adapted from National Poisons Information Service [1]

5.6.2   8–24-h Post-ingestion

If a patient presents between 8 and 24-h post-ingestion, acetylcysteine should be started immediately if the patient ingested more than 150 mg/kg paracetamol. Bloods should be taken as above to assess paracetamol concentration, liver and renal function. In this case, treatment may be stopped if the blood results do not meet the criteria. If the patient has taken less than 150 mg/kg, it is acceptable to take bloods and wait for the results to guide the treatment decision. It is unlikely that toxicity will occur if the patient has taken less than 75 mg/kg; however, that leaves a grey area with little evidence to guide management between 75 and 150 mg/kg. All treatment decisions must be taken into consideration with blood results, clinical findings and the history of the overdose. If there is any doubt or inconsistency, it is *always* safer to treat.

5.6.3   More Than 24-h Post-ingestion

If the patient presents more than 24-h post-ingestion with features of hepatotoxicity (primarily jaundice or right upper quadrant pain), the advice is to start acetylcysteine immediately and take bloods for paracetamol concentration, liver function, renal function, bicarbonate, INR and full blood count. If they have no features of hepatotoxicity, the advice is to wait for blood results to make a decision. It is more common to encounter seriously unwell patients at this stage. Consider the patient who presents as clearly jaundiced with a significantly elevated ALT and INR. By this stage the paracetamol concentration may not be substantial; however, there is clear evidence that this patient is at risk of fulminant liver failure. The priority is still to commence acetylcysteine; however, input from the liver specialists is vital as this patient may require consideration for transplant if blood tests do not improve with acetylcysteine alone. Millson et al. [8] indicate that the criteria for transplant in acute hepatic failure following paracetamol overdose includes lactic acidosis over 24-h post-overdose despite fluid resuscitation, significant coagulopathy and grades 3–4 encephalopathy. Contraindications include multiple previous episodes of self-harm and consistent suicidal ideation in the absence of established mental illness. Assessment by the liver team and the psychiatry team in unison is necessary to reach a decision. This scenario can be extremely distressing for the patient, their families and for care givers involved, particularly if the patient is familiar due to frequent presentations and has exhausted treatment options and does not meet transplant criteria.

5.6.4   Staggered and Therapeutic Excess Ingestions

Staggered paracetamol ingestions are defined as any ingestion taking place over a timeframe of more than 1-h. This could be in relation to the patient who has intentionally taken paracetamol over an hour and a half or who has taken multiple overdoses over a period of hours to days. Therapeutic excess ingestions refer to the patient who has taken over the recommended daily dosages of paracetamol in the context of symptom relief for pain or fever. This may occur because the patient was not aware of maximum doses or perhaps had been unknowingly taking multiple paracetamol containing products, for example, cocodamol, lemsip or cold and flu remedies. These scenarios are complicated, and treatment decisions again should be made in the context of the history of the overdose, clinical features and blood results.

However, the general advice is to treat with acetylcysteine. Remember that it is *always* safer to treat when the history is complicated or inconsistent.

6   Antidepressants

It is extremely common to see antidepressants used in intentional overdose, partially due to the disorders they are prescribed to treat. There are two main groups of antidepressants generally prescribed within the UK, namely, selective serotonin reuptake inhibitors (SSRIs) and tricyclic antidepressants (TCAs), both of which target monoamine (noradrenalin, serotonin and dopamine) activity in central neurons. Treatment for depression is largely based on monoamine theory which hypothesises that depression occurs due to a depletion of monoamines in the central nervous system. Thus, the treatment goal in management of depression is to increase availability of monoamines for physiological and psychological benefit. Both SSRIs and TCAs prevent the normal reuptake of monoamines whereby their biological activity would otherwise be terminated.

7   Selective Serotonin Reuptake Inhibitors

SSRIs are the first-line treatment option to manage depression and include citalopram, escitalopram, fluoxetine, paroxetine and sertraline. While generally considered less toxic than TCAs in overdose with a safer side-effect profile in therapeutic dosing, they can cause potentially fatal problems in overdose, particularly if taken with other substances.

7.1   Mechanism

These drugs act by inhibiting the reuptake of serotonin in the central nervous system, thus in overdose available serotonin may become overwhelming, causing toxicity from the serotonin itself leading to agitation and increased neuromuscular activity. In extreme doses some SSRIs can directly induce myocardial ion channel blockade leading to ventricular polarisation delays, reflected on an electrocardiogram as QRS prolongation (for sodium channels) and QT prolongation (for potassium channels). If these abnormalities are not corrected, severe arrhythmias can occur, notably ventricular fibrillation (in sodium channel blockade) and torsade de pointes (in potassium channel blockade). Central ion channel disruption can also occur manifesting clinically as seizure activity.

7.2   Clinical Features

As mentioned previously, toxidromes are clusters of features arising alongside poisoning of certain groups of drugs. SSRIs are classically associated with the serotonergic toxidrome. Most patients will have mild features including nausea, agitation, dilated pupils and tachycardia. It is important to note that features may develop or worsen, so TOXBASE® should always be consulted for advice on minimum observation periods. Citalopram is considered the most dangerous SSRI in overdose, and all presentations should be monitored for at least 12-h. More commonly QT prolongation with SSRIs, particularly citalopram, can precede torsade de pointes. Hypoglycaemia may also occur. In very large overdoses, or if SSRIs are taken with additional serotonergic drugs, there is increased chance of *serotonin syndrome*. This can be life-threatening; thus it is important to recognise this promptly.

7.3   Serotonin Syndrome/Toxicity

Serotonin syndrome is a potentially fatal outcome arising from overdose of drugs which have effects on central and peripheral serotonin receptors. It may also occur as a result of drug interactions if prescribed more than one serotonergic agent or with use of recreational drugs which have serotonergic action. It essentially occurs due to excessive serotonin available within the neural synapses. Onset of symptoms can occur within minutes or hours of ingestion. Serotonin syndrome classically comprises three groups of features:

- Altered mental state: including agitation, confusion, delirium and hallucinations to drowsiness and coma
- Neuromuscular hyperactivity: including profound shivering, tremor, bruxism, ocular clonus, inducible or spontaneous clonus and hyperreflexia
- Autonomic instability: including dilated pupils, diarrhoea, profuse sweating, flushing, tachycardia, hypertension and, most importantly, *hyperthermia*

In the more severe cases, hyperthermia is considered the most clinically significant feature. Rhabdomyolysis, renal failure and disseminated intravascular coagulopathy may develop and may indeed be a direct result of the excessive temperature.

7.4   Investigations

As with every presentation to hospital, a full set of observations is vital, as well as assessment of conscious state. A blood sugar is also important as we know that SSRI poisoning can induce hypoglycaemia. Close monitoring of temperature throughout the admission is necessary, as development of hyperthermia is the most crucial feature and requires action. Initial blood tests include U&Es and liver function tests. Additionally, a creatinine kinase (CK) is useful, particularly if pyrexia is present, which may indicate muscle damage from neuromuscular hyperactivity and potential to develop subsequent renal injury. If CK is elevated, it is always useful to repeat this in order to assess trend. A 12-lead electrocardiogram should be performed on initial assessment and then repeated serially to examine for potential developing cardiotoxicity. All cases of toxic ingestions should be monitored on telemetry until the observation period for the ingested agent is complete, as per TOXBASE®, or until features have resolved.

7.5   Management

On initial assessment, a patent airway and ventilation must be established if consciousness is reduced. It may be beneficial to give activated charcoal if presentation is within 1–2-h of ingestion, although this should be avoided if there are any airway concerns due to aspiration risk. Seizure activity can be treated with benzodiazepines. Phenytoin is contraindicated as it can contribute to potential cardiotoxicity; therefore second-line treatment for seizures unresponsive to benzodiazepines would be barbiturates. The electrocardiogram should be examined for QT prolongation, measured by use of the QT nomogram (available on TOXBASE®) which calculates level of risk of torsades de pointes by measuring against heart rate (Fig. 2). If QT prolongation exists, intravenous magnesium (8 mmol) should be administered, as a cardioprotective measure which reduces the risk of progression to torsade de pointes. The exact mechanism is unclear, but it is believed that magnesium may stabilise the cardiac membrane potential by facilitating potassium influx, thus countering the potassium channel blockade. If renal impairment occurs as a result of muscle damage, known as rhabdomyolysis, intravenous fluids should be initiated with close monitoring of renal function and electrolytes. In severe cases haemodialysis may be warranted.

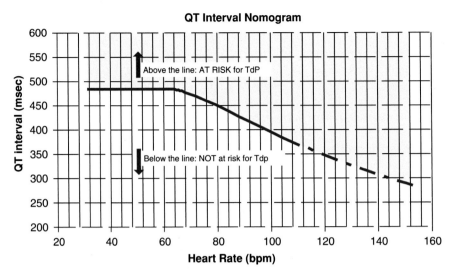

Fig. 2 QT nomogram for calculating risk of TdP. Adapted from Chan et al. [9]

7.6   Management of Serotonin Syndrome

Agitation should be managed with benzodiazepines, usually diazepam or loraze-pam. Physical restraint should be avoided as this can potentially cause further mus-cular damage. In the instance of hyperthermia, conventional cooling methods may include fans, cooled intravenous fluids and ice packs to groins/axilla. Benzodiazepines can actively assist with the cooling process and should be given regularly in con-junction with the above. As the hyperthermia is a result of excessive muscular activ-ity, traditional antipyretic therapy is not useful. Mild cases will usually resolve within 24-h using the above measures. Moderate to severe cases have anecdotally improved with use of serotonin receptor antagonists, e.g. cyproheptadine and chlor-promazine. Theoretically, these block the receptor agonism of SSRIs to allow reso-lution of features; however, there is no controlled trial evidence available.

Consider the patient who has presented to hospital with increasing agitation and confusion with an unclear history of events. Family members have reported that she has access to fluoxetine and has been known to use amphetamine. She has obvious abnormal eye movements and increased muscular tone and has spontaneous ankle clonus on examination. Her temperature is 40 °C. In this instance it is most likely she has serotonin syndrome as her symptoms are representative of all three compo-nents of the diagnostic triad of features associated with serotonin syndrome. Additionally, she is at high risk due to likely ingestion of more than one serotoner-gic agent. This case was managed with the above listed measures to no avail. If the case is severe and management is failing, then neuromuscular paralysis, intubation and ventilation in a critical care setting must be considered. There is a high risk of death associated with severe serotonin syndrome; thus early recognition and escala-tion are essential to aid full recovery.

8 Tricyclic Antidepressants (TCAs)

TCAs are commonly prescribed as second-line therapy for depression and for other indications including chronic pain. Examples include amitriptyline, nortriptyline, clomipramine and dosulepin. TCAs are more dangerous in overdose than SSRIs due to their mechanism of action and side-effect profile.

8.1 Mechanism

As well as blocking monoamine reuptake, like SSRI action, they are *nonselective* and have additional action involving histamine and acetylcholine. This results in antihistaminergic and anticholinergic effects often causing severe sedation, which may lead to compromised respiratory function and acidosis. TCAs can additionally cause sodium channel blockade in overdose, reflected as a prolonged QRS duration on the electrocardiogram. This is clinically significant as it can deteriorate to ventricular fibrillation if not detected and treated. The binding of TCAs to sodium channels is enhanced by acidosis. Seizures may arise due to central sodium channel blockade and indeed contribute to acidosis which in turn can worsen the QRS prolongation resulting in ventricular arrhythmia. Vasodilation may occur due to alpha-adrenoreceptor antagonism which can lead to secondary hypotension. Death most commonly occurs due to cardiotoxicity and convulsions; however, it is important to note that reduced consciousness and hypotension with acidosis can directly contribute to the development of these complications.

8.2 Clinical Features

Symptoms of TCA poisoning usually occur within 4-h of ingestion and primarily present as the anticholinergic toxidrome. This is characterised by dry mouth, hot dry skin, large pupils with blurred vision, tachycardia and drowsiness. Drowsiness may be further provoked by antihistamine effects. Cardiovascular and central nervous system effects may develop at variable rates dependent on amount ingested and speed of absorption. In more severe cases, central nervous system features may include brisk reflexes, coma, seizures and respiratory depression. Cardiovascular features include hypotension and QRS prolongation caused by sodium channel blockade which can in turn develop into ventricular fibrillation. In severe cases there may be a cycle of complications which may exacerbate each other. Sodium channel blockade is enhanced by hypoxia and acidosis caused by respiratory depression, thereby increasing likelihood of arrhythmias. Arrhythmias may in turn exacerbate acidosis. Hypotension may result in reduced cerebral perfusion thereby increasing risk of convulsions.

The recovery phase for TCA overdose can be additionally distressing, often led by a marked delirium. Patients may be agitated due to prolonged anticholinergic effects, particularly following significant overdoses. Classical features of this phase include incoherent, mumbling speech, ongoing dry mouth and plucking at bed clothes or clothing. Urinary retention may occur requiring a period of catheterisation.

8.3 Investigations

A full set of observations is imperative, and continuous cardiac telemetry is required until the observation period is fulfilled as per TOXBASE® if asymptomatic, or until symptoms resolve in those exhibiting clinical features. Assessment of conscious state is also vital and should be monitored frequently. Initial blood tests include U&Es and liver function tests. A 12-lead electrocardiogram should be performed on initial assessment and then repeated serially to examine for potential developing cardiotoxicity. If QRS prolongation occurs, it is useful to obtain a blood gas analysis to guide treatment. Likewise, blood gas analysis is vital if respiratory depression occurs to gauge the severity of potential acidosis. It is important to closely monitor conscious level, particularly in the earlier stages as rapid sedation within a few hours generally indicates severe poisoning.

8.4 Management

On initial assessment any airway or ventilation concerns should be addressed if consciousness is reduced. It may be beneficial to give activated charcoal if presentation is within 1 to 2-h of ingestion. Given aspiration risk, this should only be considered if the patient is maintaining their own airway. Patients who present unconscious will likely require rapid intubation, ventilation and intensivist support. These patients need careful monitoring of acid base status and correction of any arising acidosis. Patients who experience cardiac arrest require prolonged cardiopulmonary resuscitation with reports of full recovery following several hours of resuscitative measures.

A 12-lead electrocardiogram must be performed and examined for prolongation of the QRS interval (greater than 120 mmsc) (Fig. 3). This should be treated with intravenous sodium bicarbonate, and we should aim for a pH of 7.5 on blood gas analysis. Sodium bicarbonate is an alkali and the treatment regime aims for an alkalotic state. An initial bolus of 50 mmol is indicated with repeat 12-lead electrocardiogram and monitoring of serum potassium and arterial pH. Use of 8.4% sodium bicarbonate is generally advised, particularly if QRS duration is greater than 160 mmsc, but the cannula site must be closely observed for signs of extravasation. Patients who experience hypotension resistant to intravenous fluid challenges should be managed in a critical care area and may respond well to inotropes or vasopressors. Seizures again should be treated with intravenous benzodiazepines, usually diazepam or lorazepam, although close observation is required in case of arising respiratory depression which can in turn lead to acidosis and hypoxia.

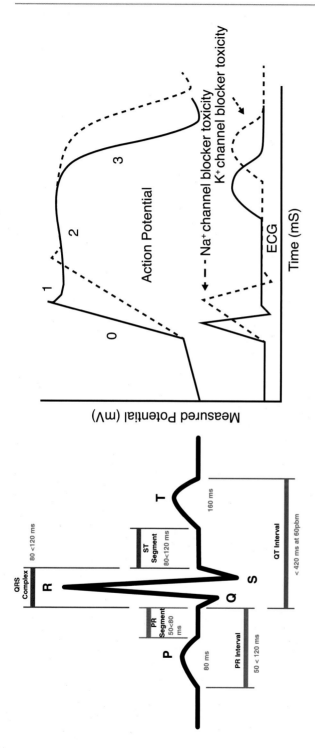

Fig. 3 Normal QRS/QT durations and cardiac action potential with corresponding ECG durations. Adapted from Bateman et al. [4] and Delk et al. [10]

Sodium bicarbonate is the key treatment for severe TCA poisoning by overwhelming sodium channel blockade and counteracting acidosis. Additionally, it has a positive effect on contractility of the myocardium so may in turn have an impact on hypotension. Intravenous lipid emulsion may offer some benefit to those with treatment resistant arrhythmias or hypotension. However, this is generally reserved for peri-arrest situations when all other more evidence-based treatments have proven futile. It works on the premise that TCAs are lipophilic (i.e. attracted to fats); therefore, they should bind to lipid emulsion introduced to the plasma in order to prevent action on target sites in the body. However, the actual mechanism is not entirely clear, and its role is yet to be fully understood.

If the patient has been severely unwell and has required intensive support through the acute phase of the overdose, it is common to experience an ongoing anticholinergic delirium. This can be distressing for the patient, their families and potentially for staff caring for them. Consider the patient who has stepped down from intensive care, whereby many patients experience disorientation and confusion due the after effect of medications used to maintain induced coma and paralysis. This combined with ongoing anticholinergic effects can be quite traumatic. They may continue to exhibit classical features of the anticholinergic toxidrome with dry mouth, urinary retention, plucking at bedclothes and mumbling incoherent speech and may suffer from frightening hallucinations or delusions. It is essential that those caring for these patients offer reassurance, both to the patient and to their families, that this is a recovery phase and will improve. These patients benefit from frequent reorientation and should be cared for in a low stimulus environment. Sedation using a long-acting benzodiazepine (e.g. diazepam) is usually effective.

9   Conclusion

Poisoning is a common emergency presentation in the UK. Patients who take intentional overdoses are often emotionally distressed and are at risk of varying harms from both the overdose itself and from their potential mental health disorders. It is vital that an atmosphere of trust is created with patients during an extremely vulnerable time. Risk assessment for potential further self-harm is important and demonstrates to the patient that their practitioners acknowledge their distress. Following an intentional overdose, all cases should be discussed with or reviewed by the mental health team. As healthcare professionals it is also imperative that we acknowledge the personal emotional cost of caring for those who have attempted suicide. Taking time between cases and clinical duties to reflect and access support from colleagues is invaluable for maintaining the ability to provide high-quality care.

Three of the most common substances used in overdose in the UK have been presented. The management of paracetamol poisoning can be complex depending on time of ingestion and whether or not the overdose was single acute or staggered over hours or days; however, there is an extremely effective antidote. The use of acetylcysteine alongside careful interpretation of the history and clinical investigations is imperative to offer the best possible outcome. Following on from paracetamol, the next most common intentional poisoning presentation is antidepressant overdose. The most regularly prescribed classes of antidepressants are SSRIs and TCAs and may present with varying degrees of severity according to amount ingested and co-ingestions of similar medicines. SSRI overdose can result in serotonin syndrome which can be potentially fatal. Early recognition of this is essential so that best supportive care can be provided. TCA overdoses are often very serious resulting in a cycle of respiratory depression, acidosis and sodium channel blockade. Sodium bicarbonate is the most effective measure in these cases, and intensivist team support in critical care areas is often necessary.

Managing acute poisonings can be complex, and there are a vast range of potential ingestions, from organic compounds and pharmaceuticals to household and industrial chemicals. Understanding management of the most common presentations is useful; however, knowing how to access the most up-to-date advice is essential. TOXBASE® should always be consulted when faced with poisoning cases to provide the most accurate and potentially life-saving support for a particularly vulnerable client group.

Learning Points
- State the three most frequently ingested products in intentional overdose and outline their presentations and management.
- Building trust with patient following overdose is essential while assessing psychological risk. Consider what mental health support you would offer and arrange.
- Consulting TOXBASE® is the best way to source the most comprehensive advice and should *always* be consulted. Outline how you would access this advice in your department.

References

1. National Poisons Information Service. TOXBASE ® © Crown Copyright 1983–2021; 2020
2. World Health Organization. Suicide prevention. WHO; 2020. https://www.who.int/health-topics/suicide#tab=tab_1
3. Hamilton I. Changing healthcare workers' attitudes to self-harm. BMJ. 2016;353:I2443. https://doi.org/10.1136/bmj.i2443.
4. Bateman ND, Jefferson RD, Thomas SHL, Thompson JP, Vale JA. Oxford desk reference: toxicology. 1st ed. Oxford: Oxford University Press; 2014. p. 194–5.
5. Sandilands EA, Morrison EE, Bateman D. Adverse reactions to intravenous acetylcysteine in paracetamol poisoning. Adverse Drug React Bull. 2016;297(1):1147–50. https://doi.org/10.1097/FAD.0000000000000015.
6. Thanacoody H, Gray A, Dear J, Coyle J, Sandilands E, Webb D, Lewis S, Eddleston M, Thomas S, Bateman D. Scottish and Newcastle antiemetic pre-treatment for paracetamol poisoning study (SNAP). BMC Pharmacol Toxicol. 2013;14(1):20. https://doi.org/10.1186/2050-6511-14-20.
7. Silvotti MLA, Juurlink DN, Garland JS, Lenga I, Poley R, Hanly LN, Thompson M. Antidote removal during haemodialysis for massive acetaminophen overdose. Clin Toxicol (Phila). 2013;51(9):855–63. https://doi.org/10.3109/15563650.2013.844824.

8. Millson C, Considine A, Cramp ME, Holt A, Hubscher S, Hutchinson J, Jones K, Leithead J, Masson S, Menon K, Mirza D, Neuberger J, Prasad R, Pratt A, Prentice W, Shepherd L, Simpson K, Thorburn D, Westbrook R, Tripathi D. Adult liver transplantation: a UK clinical guideline - part 1: pre-operation. Frontline Gastroenterol. 2019;0(1):10. https://doi.org/10.1136/flgastro-2019-101215.
9. Chan A, Isbister GK, Kirkpatrick CMJ, Dufful SB. Drug-induced QT prolongation and torsades de pointes: evaluation of a QT nomogram. QJM. 2007;100(10):609–15. https://doi.org/10.1093/qjmed/hcm072.
10. Delk C, Holstege CP, Brady WJ. Electrocardiograph abnormalities associated with poisoning. Am J Emerg Med. 2007;25:672–87. https://doi.org/10.1016/j.ajem.2006.11.038.

Printed in the United States
by Baker & Taylor Publisher Services